Nature and Wellbeing in the Digital Age

How to feel better without logging off

Sue Thomas

D1806172

ISBN-13: 978-1548291143
ISBN-10: 1548291145
2nd Edition

A note about this edition

The first edition of this book was published in digital format. For the second edition, it has been redesigned for print. Layout has been changed, some sections moved around, and page numbers added. The content has been revised in places.

About the Author

Sue Thomas's books include *Technobiophilia: nature and cyberspace*, a study of nature and technology; *Hello World: travels in virtuality*, a travelogue/memoir of life online, and the novel *Correspondence*, short-listed for the Arthur C. Clarke Science Fiction Award. She has written for a number of publications including *Orion Magazine*, *The Guardian*, and *Slate*. She was Professor of New Media at De Montfort University until 2013 and is a Visiting Fellow at Bournemouth University.

She lives by the sea in Dorset, England.

www.suethomas.net @suethomas

About 'Technobiophilia: Nature and Cyberspace'

'Technobiophilia reminds readers that we control how we use our technology—and even smartphones and screensavers can help us connect to the natural world.' (Emily Glaser, Orion Magazine)

'A useful lens for seeing where we are, who we are, and where humans, our digital creations, and the natural world are heading.' (Howard Rheingold, writer and critic)

'I'll admit it: I love tech with natural elements like wood, and I don't think I'm alone.' (Mike Elgan, Confessions of a Technobiophiliac, Computerworld)

'The book is about a powerful subliminal urge by our entire species to hang onto our connection to the natural world, as we are pulled deeper into the digital age.' (George Davis, Psychology Today)

For my family

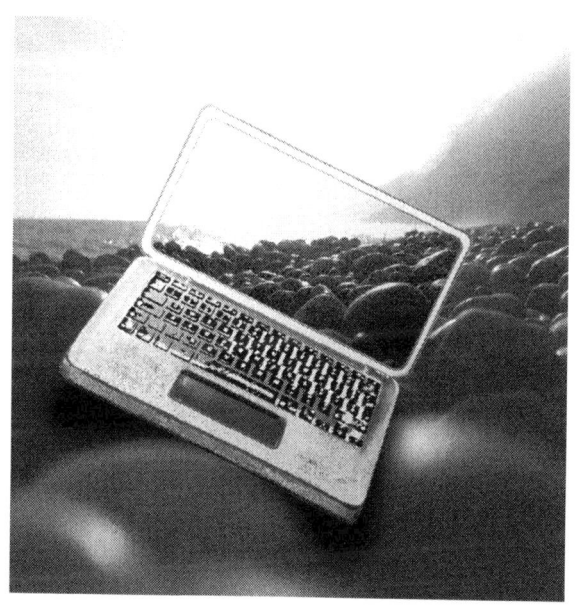

Contents

Foreword: choose more nature

Perhaps you have noticed that digital guilt has become the media's favourite way to fill an empty column or two? The smallest mention of the dangers of technology is guaranteed to make us shift uneasily as we scroll through our phones and tablets.

Remarks like this, for example, can really sting when you're doing your best just to get through the day: 'Reading Thoreau by the fire, fishing for trout, and playing chess over blackberry wine are just some of the pleasures I've found since I turned my back on tech', wrote digital detoxer Mark Boyle.[i]

Ouch! That makes me feel so inadequate, with my phone always in my pocket!

Actually, though, it doesn't have to be like that.

This little book is not about turning your back on tech or anything else. It's about re-balancing your life by choosing more nature, not less technology.

I wrote it for people who love their wired lives *and*

1

the natural world, but worry they can't have both. You can. Don't fret. Don't feel guilty. It really is possible. And there's no need to turn off your phone if you don't want to.

When my book 'Technobiophilia: nature and cyberspace' was published in 2013, it triggered an important conversation. Readers told me they loved the idea of reconnecting with the natural world without having to give up their technology, but had no idea how to go about it. They wanted a simple guide, straightforward and inspiring, with practical activities to try. Here it is.

I hope that what you find here will encourage you to add more nature to your life. Read it outdoors if you can, perhaps while you're in the park, or stretched out on the beach, or relaxing in the woods. Let it help you find your own tech/nature balance.

The book is in three parts. Part 1 explains what technobiophilia is, how I discovered it, and why it's important. Part 2 contains personal stories and research about how our digital lives connect to nature. Part 3 is a list of 50 practical activities - tips, tricks and experiments to try. Dip in anywhere you like and bookmark your favourite pages.

The contents are adapted from material written since the publication of 'Technobiophilia' and include selections from my Wired Well-being column at The Conversation, as well as other journalism, blog posts and the occasional quotation. Some parts are new and previously unpublished.

I'd love to hear your own stories and experiments. Please join me at the Digital Wellbeing Facebook Group to connect and share. https://www.facebook.com/groups/digitalwellbeing/

Author Tristan Gooley wrote that 'the joy of discovering a deep connection with nature is that it allows each of us to see each living thing, object and idea within its own intricate network.'[ii] Of course, we ourselves are part of that network too, and so therefore is technology, because we made it. There are no boundaries. Organic and inorganic, human, animal, AI - we're together on this planet, each a part of the whole.

1. How to feel better

'If you just sit and observe, you will see how restless your mind is'. (Steve Jobs)

'Nature is not a place to visit – it is home'. (Gary Snyder)

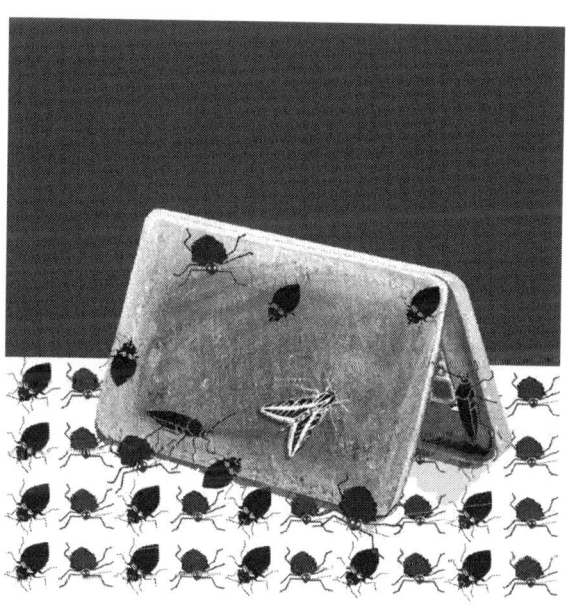

The birds in the trees

Are you concerned that you don't hear the birds in the trees? That you seldom feel the grass under your feet or the wind in your hair? That the most vivid colours in your life come from a screen?

When was the last time you sat on a beach and let the sand run between your toes? Followed footpaths across rich green meadows, inhaling the heavy scent of hawthorn hedges around their perimeter? Got lost in a wood at dusk and felt just a little bit scared?

Do you check the weather in an app, or by the way it feels on your skin?

Are you always staring at your phone and never at the sky?

If so, you're not alone.

Many people today feel divorced from the natural world. A good number blame it on their digital lives. Everything is too fast, everyone is too connected. It seems impossible to get away from your mobile, your tablet, your PC. But when you try to limit your online time, you discover something else to worry about: the fact is, you don't want to turn off your computer or leave your phone at home. You love them too much. And that's where the guilt kicks in.

But do we really need to disconnect from the internet in order to reconnect with the earth, sea and sky? I don't believe we do. That's what this book is about. Consider it an antidote to all those digital detox scare stories.

Life is changing

Our workplaces are very different from a couple of decades ago, even probably just one decade ago. More of us are part-time, freelance, or employed on zero hours contracts. Many of us no longer work in factories, offices or shops, but at home in the kitchen, nomadically between cafes, libraries and gyms with free wifi, or in specially-designed collaborative offices created for self-employed start-ups. Quite a few of those spaces were repurposed from their earlier incarnations as banks, retail outlets and warehouses after they became defunct in the new economy. Indeed, some companies are now adopting similar kinds of free-wheeling models where employees can work flexibly at home or on the road.

Our homes are often different too. We're no longer expecting to buy our first house any time soon. Instead, we're staying with extended family for longer, or renting a flat, or even perpetually travelling the world as digital nomads. Some of us are employed but homeless. Most of us don't have a place to plant and grow things. Our nearest patch of green may be a communal garden we're not allowed to tend, or a park the council can no longer afford to take care of. Most of us are urban. The minority who live in rural areas have better access to the outdoors but may be trapped there by lack of transport and and resources – problems which make the pleasures of nature the least of their concerns.

In the heart of all this difficulty, attention to

wellbeing seems like a luxury most can barely afford financially, practically, or emotionally. But think of it another way. Depending on how you do it, connecting with nature can be one of the least expensive luxuries. And there are few experiences more restorative and rewarding. So can you find a way to make time for it in your digital life?

We know nature is good for us

The wonderful sensations of the sun warming our skin or the icy kiss of snowflakes landing on our cheeks need no explanation. They remind us that we're alive, part of the planet we live on. Our DNA contains the history of the Earth and we're all, as cosmologist Carl Sagan said, made of starstuff. We know it in our bones.

Yet, for several millennia we've worked to build a world designed to disconnect us from nature. We've made structures and materials to protect us from it; found ways to farm and cook its plants and animals; invented the wheel, stories, writing, music, pictures, and all kinds of manufacturing and processing methods. We've built ships, cars, aeroplanes, and space rockets. And, in the last few decades, we built the internet. Then we added Facebook, Twitter, YouTube, Microsoft Word and, the very devil incarnate, the smartphone. So, now what?

The rift

Some fear we've gone too far and we'll soon be overcome by our own technology. They think that whether we're subsumed into a world run by robots, or superseded by superior intelligences, or simply blown up by our own stupidity… whatever it is, we've stepped over the line and will eventually pay the price.

That's certainly possible. But it's not a reason to stop everything and try to turn back the tide because it's also conceivable that, far from separating us from the natural world, our phones, smart watches, tablets and PCs can bring us closer to it. Perhaps they will even help heal the rift between us and our planet.

But this book is not about futuristic inventions which could save the world. Its proposal is much simpler than that. It merely suggests that we stop wasting time hating technology and redirect that energy towards loving nature instead.

Many people have already discovered that virtual encounters with nature can be extremely powerful. Video games can transport us into wild yet often healing environments and even the humblest screen saver picture can bring calm to a moment of calm to a stressful day.

For example, while you agonise over whether you need a digital detox, thousand of amateur farmers in windowless offices around the world are taking time out from a stressful day at the keyboard to tend their virtual tomato plants in FarmVille. Elsewhere, Grand Theft Auto players explore gorgeous wild landscapes lit with a compelling natural beauty in real uncanny valleys. And 350 million photos are posted on Facebook every day.

How many of those are of our own gardens and daily walks? Quite a few, I suspect.

That's the way of our digital lives today. But, remember, we're only at the beginning. The wired world is in its infancy and there's a lot to learn. We're still taking baby steps and sometimes we stumble and trip, but let us not forget that the internet has brought us to the cusp of something amazing. We can't help but embrace it, but we must make sure that we don't lose touch with nature in the process.

The dancer and craftsman Paulus Berensohn once said of his complex and dynamic work 'it is not a way of making a living, it is a way of making a life'. It's the same with digital technology. We use it for making a living, yes, but we also use it for making a life.

It took me a long time to realise that.

I don't live as well as I should

In the last twenty years or so there have been

very few days when I've not connected to the World Wide Web. I was born into one of the first generations to encounter the world through a TV screen, and I discovered the internet when I was 43. I've been online for a third of my life.

In the early days, I logged on to the music of a dial-up modem, a tune which still thrills me whenever I hear it. It sounded like the revving of an aeroplane before take-off, or the engine of a car gathering speed. I couldn't wait for the low vibrating dongg-dongg-dongg of the hardware handshake followed by a breathless pause until you knew for certain that you were online. In those days, connections were so fragile that logging on felt like leaping across a precipice and just hoping the other side would take your weight.

As soon as I discovered cyberspace I knew it would become my muse, and so it has proved. It felt like the home of my heart, the place where I could really be me, my own personal geography. I've written about it ever since. It has given me a career as a writer and academic, but it was only

14

while researching my most recent book, 'Technobiophilia: nature and cyberspace', that I realised I needed to get my act together.

I came to understand that I don't get outside enough; I don't connect with nature enough; I don't even touch the world enough. My gaze is always on a screen. My thoughts are always in cyberspace.

I still love my wired life and I'm not prepared to give it up, but I do have questions. Where are we headed? What should we be doing to ensure that our digital lives are healthy, mindful and productive? How can I connect to my body and to the world without breaking up with technology? I think I've begun to find some answers, but there's still a lot of work to do.

Let us make a start in wild nature, hiking in the Californian Sierras alongside the legendary John Muir.

Heading for the hills

John Muir was born in 1838 in the Scottish town of Dunbar. When he was eleven his family emigrated to the USA but it wasn't until his thirties that he got to know the mountains of California and fell in love with their dramatic landscapes. He told many colourful stories about his adventures in the High Sierras and his passionate advocacy for the wild is still much admired today.

Muir regularly voiced his contempt for urban life. For example, one day he was out hiking on his own when he had a minor accident. He fell some distance down a mountainside, landed in a clump of spiny chaparral bushes, and was briefly knocked unconscious. Later, he wrote that when he came round he blamed his fall on spending too much time in the city (he lived in San Francisco with his family when he wasn't out hiking). That, he told himself, 'is what you get by intercourse with stupid town stairs, and dead pavements.' At least, however, the spill had properly woken him up and

16

he felt 'confident that the last of the town fog had been shaken from both head and feet'.

As environmentalist and author George Monbiot wrote, 'We head for the hills to escape the order and control that sometimes seem to crush the breath out of us.' We often blame the city, that 'town fog' as Muir called it, for the 'unnatural' lives we lead. These days we don't accuse new-fangled technologies like stairs and pavements of causing our plight, but instead blame cars, planes and TVs. More recently, of course, the internet has leapt to the top of the culpability list.

It's almost five decades since 1969, when the first two nodes of what was then called Arpanet were connected, but the internet still has the capacity to make us anxious. We know there's a problem because so many people feel overwhelmed by their digital lives. In a culture where to be disconnected increasingly means to be disenfranchised, it's not surprising that we dream about breaking away and starting a new life off the grid (although maybe not this week).

17

Threading through this general discomfiture is the fear that technology has literally and irrevocably cast us out of The Garden. Many influential voices have been raised to support that idea. In 1996, eco-philosopher David Abram cautioned that we allow technology to shut us off from the natural world[iii]. Two years later, farmer and writer Wendell Berry complained 'I do not see that computers are bringing us one step nearer to anything that does matter to me: peace, economic justice, ecological health, political honesty, family and community stability, good work.'[iv]

Today, the internet-anxiety industry thrives on headlines like '10 Ways The Internet Is Destroying You', 'Too Much Internet Is Bad For Your Brain' and, the most potent variety of all, 'The Internet Can Be Bad For Children's Mental Health' (note the cautious 'can' hidden inside that sentence). The net, and its offspring the World Wide Web, have both brought many changes to the way we connect and interact with each other, but have they really shut us off from the natural world?

A battle for our digital souls

A parent of two teenagers once told me that her family are all keen users of technology and she has absolutely no doubts about the benefits of wired life. But, Liz[v] added sadly, they didn't pay attention to nature as often as they might.

'We all have bikes that no one rides, we have woods nearby that we seldom walk in, even a bog we visit maybe once a year and it's just down the road! Sometimes, it seems a life half lived'.

She makes sure they spend family holidays playing at the beach or exploring the forest. 'They discover so many things,' she told me. 'You can hear the sense of wonder in their voices'.

Back home again, she tries to balance her children's screen time with going outdoors. It's there, she believes, that stolen minutes spent walking in the sunshine or bird-watching in the local churchyard 'feed the spirit all week'.

Is she being sentimental? Or is her family

seriously missing out? There's certainly research to support her concern, and many of us know from personal experience that being out in nature makes us feel vital and alive. According to the World Health Organisation, for example, 'the evidence shows that urban green space has health benefits, particularly for economically deprived communities, children, pregnant women and senior citizens'. WHO is committed to 'provide each child with access to healthy and safe environments and settings of daily life in which they can walk and cycle to kindergartens and schools, and to green spaces in which to play and undertake physical activity, by 2020'.[vi]

Technology, meanwhile, is suspected of damaging us in a multitude of ways which are often presented in poorly researched but sensational news stories. As I write this, the Huffington Post has a headline 'Reading on a screen before bed might be killing you'[vii] (note the 'might'). The piece describes an experiment with just 12 participants over 2 weeks – hardly enough evidence to make any kind of claim. Yet this kind of scare-mongering gets much more coverage than more positive views on the subject.

Most of us have an intuitive appreciation of the benefits of a more 'natural' life. For example, when a stressed-out friend sighs 'I need to get back to nature for a while', we immediately understand what they mean. It's a longing for a less complicated day-to-day, one which takes them away from the oppressiveness of modern life with its 'town fog' of streets, traffic, noise, email, phones and always-on mentality. They want, to use a technological metaphor, to press their own personal reset button.

Many of us see ourselves as hapless victims caught in a battle for our digital souls. We worry whether we should exercise more self-control, close down the computer and take a walk outdoors. Get back to nature with a digital detox, or turn off the internet for the weekend and observe an electronic Sabbath. We wonder how better life might be if we could only summon the willpower to leave our phones at home and enjoy nature in the (offline) raw.

The anxiety grows even stronger when we look at our children and their dwindling interactions with the outdoors. No matter how hard we try, our busy lifestyles mean ever-reducing leisure hours and with them go many opportunities for wild time.

I worry too

I confess that I've been feeling something of this anxiety myself. Do I pay enough attention to feeding my spirit?

My life has been dominated by cyberspace for many years now. I love being out in the wilds of the internet, exploring, learning, connecting. I'm at home there. But I'm starting to realise that in my passion for virtuality I've become separated from what some people call 'real life'; from what's going on in the fields, forests, skies, rivers and oceans.

When reality finally hit, around about 2011, I saw what was missing from my life. It was that muddy, aromatic, unpredictable environment to be found not just in the countryside but also threaded through our everyday experience. Wild and cultivated, nature is scattered through cities, along footpaths and motorways, in gardens, on balconies, in parks, beside water. It's everywhere, but often I don't notice it at all.

And that takes me back to technobiophilia, and how I discovered it.

Nature is on our screens

In 2004 I had a question - why do we use nature metaphors to describe cyberspace? After all, it's not even real, let alone physical. Yet look at all those terms - fields, webs, clouds, streams, rivers, trails, paths, torrents and islands; flora such as apples, blackberries, trees, roots and branches, and fauna including spiders, viruses, worms, pythons, lynxes, gophers, not to mention the ubiquitous bug and mouse. As Wired magazine founder Kevin Kelly once said, 'the web smells like life'.

I interviewed engineers, authors and academics. I read up on the history of the net; surfed the web, scoured scholarly papers, and poked about inside programming languages, but nowhere could I find anything to explain why we visualise this most abstract of places in such a physical way. My training as an English and History specialist with a smattering of computing meant that I tended to approach research from the humanities side of things, but gradually I found myself sliding towards the unknown territories of scientific enquiry.

Then one day I was reading a paper about the psychology of nature when I came across a word which was new to me – biophilia. Curious, I followed the footnotes and found myself at a book of the same name. It was written by a biologist I had never heard of at the time but who, I later discovered, is one of the most visionary scientists of our age - Edward O. Wilson.

And then it all fell into place.

Biophilia: the hidden programme

One day in 1974, E.O. Wilson was working in a shady glade in the heart of a tropical forest in Surinam, where he was researching the behaviours of ants. Suddenly, he was overcome by a feeling of intense revelation as he became aware, as never before, that he was an outsider in that place.

Years later he wrote, 'the uncounted products of evolution were gathered there for purposes having nothing to do with me'.[viii] At that moment he understood that there in the forest, surrounded by numerous species with their hugely varied and ancient genetic histories, his presence was completely inconsequential. And far from being frightened by this realisation, he felt strangely calmed by it.

It would be ten years before Wilson finally distilled his impressions into the concept of *biophilia*, which he defined as 'an innate attraction to life and lifelike processes'.

Biophilia is now widely understood as the impulse

that attracts us to the outdoors, to plant and animal life, to the green of the forests and to the blue of skies, lakes, rivers and oceans. It's the driving force behind our hunger for nature and probably holds the secret of its therapeutic qualities.

How biophilia works

'What is it exactly that binds us so closely to living things'? wrote Wilson. In his book 'Biophilia', he explains his theory that, as humans evolved, we survived by attuning to our surroundings and 'reading' the behaviours of creatures and landscapes around us. In those very early times, these skills were crucial to our survival. We needed to to be able to interpret sounds and smells, know what to do when the weather changed, and find food and shelter at desperate moments. Failure to do so could mean the difference between life and death.

Even in today's modern world we still retain that sensitivity. No matter how urban our lifestyle, how domesticated our day-to-day, an encounter with nature can momentarily stop us in our tracks. This is because, says Wilson, biophilia was genetically encoded inside the earliest humans as we struggled to survive in the wild. Today, our everyday lives are somewhat less dependent upon our physical environs, at least in the short term, but biophilia remains coded into human memory.

Moreover, Wilson thinks it might even lie dormant for long periods until something triggers it back into the forefront of our unconscious minds. An encounter with an animal, a visit to the countryside, even just the scent of a flower, can plunge us back into that ancient biophilic sensorium. In that moment, we sense a glimmer of the wild as we once knew it and suddenly we're reconnected with our ancient self. The effect might be fleetingly brief, or it can lead to a profound and life-changing moment.

George Monbiot echoes the concept of biophilia in his belief that we possess a 'ghost psyche', 'a set of capacities that helped secure our survival in more dangerous times' which today, he thinks, has become vestigial. He pictures it as 'a seam of intense emotion, buried so deeply in our minds that we can seldom find it'.[ix]

Biophilia may be invisible and hard to quantify but it's extremely powerful. You might sniff a strawberry and activate an ancient yet thrilling buzz of foraging for your daily meal. Watch a spider run across the floor and feel a surge of biophobia in your brain which heralds, not the love of nature, but a fear of it which was deeply encoded in your subconscious at an evolutionary moment when sleeping on the ground was the only option.

It's likely, but not yet proven, that humans probably have a partly genetic predisposition to biophobia. We may respond fearfully to certain living things (most notably spiders, snakes and bugs) and also to some natural situations which might contain hidden dangers and be difficult to escape from. Just as we're attracted to some kinds of animals and drawn to particular places, we can equally be repelled by others, often for sound

28

survival reasons.

Think of biophilia as a hidden programme constantly running in the background of your consciousness. Hear a blackbird sing? See that blue sky? Feel the tide running between your toes? Biophilia.

Environmental psychology

My discovery of biophilia led me to environmental psychology, an area entirely new to me. In the subject journals I discovered many research projects which have measured, assessed and evaluated the effects of human exposure to the natural world.

For example, in 1986, healthcare design researcher Roger Ulrich showed photographic slides to test subjects and concluded that slides of 'unspectacular' scenes of nature elicited an increase in positive mood, while slides of urban areas produced a decline in mood. He reported that scenes of nature, particularly those depicting water, had a beneficial influence on participants.[x] In 1989, psychologists Rachel and Stephen Kaplan found that mental fatigue could be alleviated, and levels of concentration improved, by spending more time in nature or even just from viewing nature.[xi] And Japanese researchers have found measurable benefits in patients who have spent time 'forest bathing'. This involves spending periods of time in a forest under certain kinds of conditions, and has led to improvements of blood glucose levels, mood, stress, and even (reportedly) cancer.[xii]

But as I read more about environmental psychology research, I noticed something which was evident but seldom mentioned - much of it took place, not outdoors amongst in real nature, but indoors by way of pictures, photographs and videos, as in two of the three projects described above. This approach allowed researchers to test under controlled conditions, of course, but it meant that some of the most frequently cited experiments proving the beneficial effects of nature are actually proving the benefits, not of being outside on grass or amongst trees and flowers, but of viewing images of them through a window, in a picture, *or even on a screen.*

A *screen*? Could this also apply to computers? I began to search for similar research conducted with nature viewed on computer screens but drew a blank. In fact, most of the projects which underpin this area of study were conducted in the nineteen eighties and nineties, when computers were not yet ubiquitous.

I think there was a cultural barrier in play too. It's a gross assumption, I know, but I'm guessing that the kinds of people working on nature and the outdoors in those years probably had very different priorities from those of the geeks who were busy, at the same time, inventing cyberculture in rarefied research institutions and teenage bedrooms. For example, in 1984, the year Wilson published 'Biophilia', cyberpunks and hackers were queuing up to read William Gibson's relentlessly urban science fiction novel 'Neuromancer', especially noteworthy because it coined a new word – 'cyberspace'. It was a case of two worlds which were definitely not colliding.

Furthermore, I could find no research into the psychological impact of looking at nature images on computers or phones of any kind. There's plenty of psychological research into computer use, but virtually none into the connections between environmental psychology and screen-based nature imagery. (For one example, see Deltcho Valtchanov later in this book). I realised that this was an entirely new field, and I seemed to be about the only person in it.

I began to understand how, for example, a screensaver of a beautiful waterfall cascading across an office worker's computer screen can provide an important moment of time out during the business day. And I saw how, as we explored the new landscapes of cyberspace, we used terms drawn from the language of our earliest beginnings to name it and describe the experiences we were having there. Suddenly it all made sense, and biophilia was the key.

Technobiophilia

If such powerful results could be obtained by comparatively traditional methods, would they not also apply to other kinds of screens? And did it make a difference, I wondered, whether the screen was a video, commonly used in many of the tests I had read about, or a computer screen-saver, or a photo shared on Facebook, or an event live-streamed online? I didn't see how it could possibly matter. The media are visually the same. The only difference lies in the platforms upon which they are delivered.

This was quite a surprise, and one with far-reaching consequences. I drew the conclusion that, in the light of that evidence I had seen, it makes sense that a trip to the mountains in Grand Theft Auto, or the sight of beautiful beach on your screen wallpaper, or the process of 'liking' a photo of a sunset shared on Twitter, could have the same kinds of beneficial effects as if they were actual physical encounters with nature.

I've called this phenomenon 'technobiophilia'. The term builds upon E.O Wilson's original definition by adding on just five more words. Whilst he described biophilia as 'the innate attraction to life and lifelike processes', I defined technobiophilia as **'the innate attraction to life and lifelike processes *as they appear in technology'*.**

Technobiophilic practices, objects and devices have one or more of the following features:

- they connect our lives in nature with our lives in the digital

- they contribute to wellbeing via a tech/nature balance

- and they support future biodiversity as technology and nature move closer together.

Technobiophilia has revolutionised the way I think about my digital life. It has helped me to understand that all those sunsets we share on

34

Facebook, the hours we spend roaming forests and deserts in video games, the heart-stopping adventures we enjoy in virtual reality, even the animated jellyfish floating hypnotically across our screensavers, are not random. We've chosen them, subconsciously or not, to help us relax, to make us feel good, and to soothe our connected minds.

Indeed, they are the reason we feel better without logging off.

Getting rid of the guilt

We complain that our devices make us stressed out, but how much of that stress is caused by feeling guilty that we want them in the first place?

You may have noticed that quite a lucrative industry has grown up around device-guilt. You could spend a fair bit of cash on therapists who promise to wean you away from your mobile phone. You can buy apps which lock you out of your own computer, stop you from getting to your email, and limit the amount of time you spend on Facebook.

Is that what you want?

I would like to propose a different way. Instead of there being an 'either/or' around nature and technology, what if there was just an 'and'? You can go for a bike ride *and* take your phone. You can take a walk *and* use your digital camera. You can harvest your virtual crops in FarmVille in the morning *and* dig your real garden in the afternoon.

Recently I heard an interview with a therapist who advised that gradually building up the amount of time you spend away from your smartphone will reduce your stress. It sounds good, but does it work? I know plenty of people whose stress levels increase exponentially when they can't be contacted. The same woman also advised reducing the time you look at your phone and increasing instead the time you spend reading a book. Why, in all the stars, is reading on paper better than reading on a phone?

Let us try it another way.

Forget about your online time. Think instead about your nature time, what some researchers have called your 'daily dose' of nature. Can you increase it? Can you be mindful enough to fully absorb and enjoy it? If you can manage your contact with nature, both real and virtual, you might find that your stress is reduced and so, with luck, is your device-guilt.

You're in control, not your phone

We're living in a period of what futurist Alvin Toffler called 'future shock'. He described it as undergoing too much change in too short a period of time. It's not surprising that digital technologies make us feel helpless sometimes, or that our natural instinct is to resist.

But consider this. The digital world is indeed new, but it's no different from many other future shocks endured in the past. Plato thought the invention of writing was a dangerous substitution for the common practice of simply remembering things. 'It will implant forgetfulness in their souls' and lead, he said, to 'men filled, not with wisdom, but with the conceit of wisdom.' That's to say, just being able to read a paragraph doesn't mean you're clever enough to understand it.

For Plato, writing was problematic. In 19th century England, it was the act of reading that became the enemy, especially when it concerned the reading of novels. It was believed that the imaginary worlds inhabited by fiction readers tempted them to try to take their fantasies 'into the real'. Plus, fiction was thought to increase indolence.[xiii] Relaxing with a novel, which these days is seen as an innocent comfort, was considered a very undesirable act in Victorian times.

Today, both of these fears are summed up in Baroness Susan Greenfield's call to action: 'Today's screen technologies create environments that could alter how we process information, the degree to which we take risks, how we socialise and empathise with others and even, how we view our own identity.'[xiv] Actually, all learning alters our brains and our behaviours, because that's how learning works, whether it's learning how to wash your face or connect to a wifi signal.

I believe we should temper our fear of screens and instead look for calmer, more balanced ways to live with technology. Let us choose a life for ourselves wherein the digital is smoothly integrated into the day to day. You can turn it off when you want to, and you can turn it on when you want to. It's up to you. Select a daily dose of nature and blend it into your wired life. Or choose a daily dose of digital and blend into your natureful life.

It's your decision. You are in control, not your smartphone.

You really can blend nature and wellbeing into your digital life. In Part 2, I expand upon why and how this can work, and in Part 3 there are 50 practical activities to try for yourself.

2. Rediscovering

'The real voyage of discovery consists not in making new landscapes but in having new eyes.'
(Marcel Proust)

'Take time to listen and talk about the voices of the earth and what they mean - the majestic voice of thunder, the winds, the sound of surf or flowing streams.' (Rachel Carson)

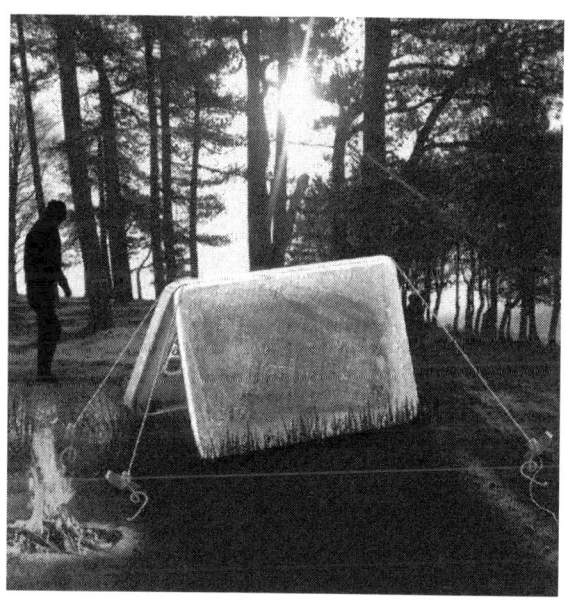

Just looking at nature is good for you

One afternoon about ten years ago, I was at San Francisco International Airport waiting for a flight to Vancouver, when I noticed that a man sitting close by had the most gorgeous photograph of a forest on his laptop screen. He wasn't particularly looking at it, it was just right there in front of him. A bright green forest, perched on his knees.

As I peered surreptitiously over his shoulder, I was reminded of how many of us adorn our hi-tech equipment with images of natural scenes, and of how this is reinforced by the default pictures provided by computer and mobile phone manufacturers. The more sophisticated our plastic and metal hardware becomes, the more we use it to take us back to nature.

When I give talks about how our love of nature intertwines with our love of technology, I often ask the audience to put up their hands if they have a nature photo on their screensavers or wallpapers. Usually, at least half of them do. I'm not surprised

43

by that. Environmental psychology has shown over and over again that just looking at pictures of nature such as photos, paintings, and videos can slow the heartbeat and reduce stress and anxiety. Of course, nothing beats the real thing, but images come a very close second.

In 1971, healthcare design expert Roger Ulrich conducted a now famous research project[xv] involving patients recovering from gall bladder surgery. It showed that patients placed in a ward with a window view of some fairly ordinary trees required less pain relief and recovered faster than similar patients in a ward where the windows looked out onto brick walls.

Other researchers developed variations of Ulrich's research. In 1984, for example, psychiatrist Aaron Katcher and his team at the University of Pennsylvania set up an experiment in the busy waiting room of a dentist's office. On some days, before the surgery opened, the researchers installed an aquarium full of fish. On other days they took it away. They measured the patients' anxiety in both environments, and the results were very clear. On aquarium days, patients were less anxious in the waiting room and (rather chillingly, perhaps) more compliant during treatment.[xvi]

A further group of researchers in a different dentist's office used a large nature mural instead of an aquarium and got similar results. Another experiment found that stressed blood donors experienced lowered blood pressure and pulse rates while sitting in a room where a videotape of a nature scene was playing on TV. The general conclusion was that visual exposure to nature not only diminishes patient stress but can also reduce physical pain.

In 1986, Ulrich set up an experiment using video. 120 subjects first viewed a stressful movie, then watched videos filmed in either natural or urban settings. Using a battery of physiological tests, their stress levels were obtained before and after watching the movie. The results showed that subjects who were exposed to the nature videos

45

recovered from the stress of the movie faster and more completely than those who had viewed videos of urban environments. The researchers concluded that the restorative influence of nature had helped the nature video watchers shift towards a more positive emotional state whilst also undergoing measurable positive changes in their levels of physiological activity.[xvii]

These kinds of tests have been repeated numerous times around the world in offices, schools, hospitals and prisons, always with similar results. This work has had a powerful and transformational impact on architectural and interior design.

It's worth noting that most of this research took place before the World Wide Web was born, but it contains many lessons for today's digital world.

Gazing at clouds

In 2009, the Norwegian public broadcaster NRK started experimenting with live, slow-paced TV shows. First they live streamed a day of sheep shearing, then a seven-hour train journey across the country from east to west. This was followed by a six-day trip by cruise ship from south to north, then by twelve hours of knitting.

In 2016 they broadcast a live stream of Saltstraumen, the world's strongest tidal current. Situated about 80km north of the Arctic circle, Saltstraumen is a narrow strait linking two fjords where sea water can flow through at speeds of up to 25mph, creating complicated and beautiful marine maelstroms.

'People will experience the calm of watching the current,' said one of the presenters. And they did. Some viewers gazed at the ebb and flow of the sea for the full twelve hours.

Psychologists Rachel and Stephen Kaplan showed that not only does pleasurable contact with nature aid recovery from mental fatigue, but the aesthetic qualities of the patterns and rhythms of the natural world induce a sense of both mystery and organisation.

They identified two related behaviours they called 'soft' and 'hard' fascination. Examples of soft fascination include gazing at clouds drifting by, watching birds and animals, and listening to the sounds of nature. Such activities relax the mind but still leave time for gentle thought and reflection. Hard fascination, on the other hand, involves very intense attention, demanding complete concentration and leaving little time for thinking things over. It can be found in a multitude of behaviours, from doing a practical task to getting a spreadsheet to balance or writing an important document.

Both types of fascination are so absorbing that they draw our minds away for a short while and allow other parts of the brain to rest. The Kaplans learned that time spent in nature can have a similar effect by helping to clear our heads and discard mental clutter. A walk in the garden or on the beach helps us refocus that ability to pay attention which is so vital to our daily cognitive functioning, whilst also providing moments of mental quiet.

There was one outcome of their investigations, however, which surprised them. Some participants reported that time spent in nature allowed them an opportunity to reflect, reassess and review personal priorities. This was a result, the Kaplans reported, which they were not looking for and would never have suspected had it not emerged so clearly in their data. They came to see it as akin to entering the sacred grove found in many religions: a quiet forest clearing where sunlight pierces the tall trees and the only sounds are birdsong and the whispering of leaves in the gentle breeze. A space to think.

Take a walk in the woods

Some days when I need a little head-space, I log in to the virtual world of Second Life and go straight to Chakryn Forest. Clothed in an avatar which looks just like me (black top and trousers, white hair), I saunter between giant sequoias, taking care not to trip over the gnarly exposed roots which connect them. Eventually, I settle quietly on a grassy hummock beside a fast-running stream and do a little forest bathing.

On other days, a physical trip to a nearby forest feels like the best option. The New Forest in Dorset, England, is two hundred square miles of woodland and heath which begins just a fifteen-minute drive from my home. I can step into a grove of aromatic pines dripping with rain and make my way through the trees between damp fairy rings of fungi and the muddy hoof marks of wild forest ponies until I find a dry spot beside a stream which looks a little less dramatic than the virtual one in Chakryn Forest. There, too, I can enjoy an hour or so of forest bathing.

Forest bathing, or 'shinrin-yoku', has been a popular activity in Japan for many years. Lately it has attracted a lot of international attention because it seems to provide measurable levels of relaxation and reduce stress.

The idea is that, simply by spending time in a

forest, the visitor breathes in volatile substances, called phytoncides, which are produced by the trees and believed to have a number of therapeutic effects ranging from stress reduction to cancer prevention. The species of tree which seems to provide the most beneficial effects is a type of Japanese pine, but they can be found in broadleaf forests too. The therapy is not just about being amongst the trees but also includes the sensory pleasures of the scenery itself, the smell of wood, the feel of touching bark and leaves, and the sound of running streams and rustling underfoot.

Dr Qing Li, a professor at Nippon Medical School and president of the Society of Forest Medicine, advises that whilst forest bathing it's not important to do heavy physical exercise, but that rather one should enjoy the forest through the five senses: 'the murmuring of a stream, birds singing, green colour, fragrance of the forest, eat some foods from the forest and just touch the trees'. [xviii]

Needless to say, forest bathing can't (yet) be fully undertaken in a digital environment deprived of smell and touch, so I can't get the full shinrin-yoku experience in Second Life. But it comes a worthy second.

Dr Li recommends that 'If you take whole day forest bathing, it is better to stay in forest for about 4 hours and walk about 5 kilometres. If you take a half day forest bathing, it is better to stay in forest for about 2 hours and walk about 2.5 kilometres'.

Like shinrin-yoku practitioners, some Western researchers are interested in finding the correct 'dose' of nature. In 2014, scholars at the Universities of Illinois at Urbana–Champaign and Hong Kong used a carefully-designed experiment to find out whether it's more calming to view a single tree or a number of trees. [xix]

They put 160 participants through a series of tests designed to induce psychological stress. The tests included 3 minutes to prepare a 5-minute public speech, giving that speech, and doing a 5-minute mental arithmetic task in front of two interviewers and a video camera. To increase stress levels, participants were told that their performance would be recorded and assessed later, but actually no video recording was made. During the tests, they were asked to report on their stress levels several times.

After their levels of stress were raised, participants viewed specially recorded 6-minute videos of varying kinds of landscapes, then undertook the tests again. After that they were given 15 minutes to write about how they had felt during the experiment. The researchers analysed the writing to evaluate the subjects' stress levels and found an interesting correlation between recovery from stress and density of tree cover. At the lowest level of tree density, only 41% of participants reported a calming effect, but as tree cover density reached 36%, more than 90% of participants reported a stress recovery experience.

The team concluded that there's 'a positive, linear association between the density of urban street trees and self-reported stress recovery'. In other words, if you're feeling stressed, hang out in a place where there are lots of trees, and you'll probably be able to relax.

Did you notice that the research described above used only videos of trees, not real trees? This prevalence of videos acting as substitutes for real nature in environmental psychology research once again prompts the question - if videos, why not screensavers? Or computer games? Or virtual reality?

Green offices increase productivity

It's traditional to have a houseplant in the office. Usually just the one, brought in years ago by some long-gone colleague. It's probably a spider plant, surviving against the odds on a dusty windowsill above a radiator and impervious to neglect. If you need to stretch your legs, you might wander over to water it. Perhaps you'll even trim off the dead leaves now and again. But generally nobody cares about it, and certainly no-one ever spends time admiring it.

54

That's all changing. Big corporations are investing huge amounts in biophilic workplaces featuring natural materials like plants, stones, wood, and water. Look out for walls festooned with hanging planters, indoor waterfalls, and stony zen gardens. Companies aren't doing this because it's cosy, but because there's increasing evidence that biophilic workplaces make employees happier and therefore more productive.

There's still a long way to go, however, before that straggling spider plant gets the care and attention it deserves.

A 2015 study by Human Spaces[xx] of 7,600 office-based employees from 16 countries found that 58% of respondents had no plants and 47% had no natural light in the office. Almost a fifth reported that there were no natural elements present in their workplace at all and a quarter said they had no sense of light and space there. Just under half of the sample had felt stressed in their workplace within the last three months. When researchers asked workers what they most wanted to see in their offices, they said:

- Natural light (44%)
- Indoor plants (20%)
- Quiet working space (19%)
- View of the sea (17%)
- Bright colours (15%)

How does your workplace compare?

A year before the Human Spaces study, The World Green Building Council produced a lengthy report on the many benefits of applying biophilic principles to the workplace. Here are just three of the many examples it cites[xxi]:

- A study of workers in a Californian call centre found that having a better view out of a window was consistently associated with better overall performance: workers were found to process calls 7% to 12% faster.

- Computer programmers with views spent

15% more time on their primary task, while equivalent workers without views spent 15% more time talking on the phone or to one another.

- The impact of indoor planting was tested at the Winterswijk Tax Office in the Netherlands in 2001. The study was carried out using a control group (without plants) and a test group (with plants) in comparable areas of the building. The most significant findings of the study included improvements in air quality (both measured and perceived by the employees) and improvements in productivity. Staff processed their work more efficiently and concentration improved, particularly in those working at computer terminals, where plants were present.

Does your employer have a Health and Wellbeing Officer yet? If not, it may soon appoint one. At the very minimum, they will advise that workplaces should contain plenty of natural light and indoor plants, and that windows look out onto green spaces.

Walking in nature helps you think

When I'm stuck on a writing problem I can't fix, or have an intractable personal anxiety, or even just feel strung out for no obvious reason, I take a walk on the beach or in a local park near my home. Occasionally I get into the car and drive to the forest, or some other stretch of green or blue.

I can't count the number of times this has resulted in an aha moment. Aha! I suddenly know how to do it! Aha! Why am I worrying about that? Aha! So that's what's eating at me!

Henri Poincaré was a pioneering mathematician with a deep interest in creativity and subliminal thought. He was just one of many thinkers who have solved problems by going for a walk and allowing their minds to wander too (mind-wandering is an old concept which has become quite a thing lately – Google it). On one occasion, Poincaré had failed to resolve some arithmetic problems so, he later explained,

'Disgusted with my failure, I went to spend a few days at the seaside and thought of something else. One morning, walking on the bluff, the idea came to me, with just the same characteristics of brevity, suddenness and immediate certainty, that the arithmetic transformations of indefinite ternary quadratic forms were identical with those of non-Euclidian geometry.[xxii]

I've no idea what he's talking about, but clearly it was the walk on the bluffs that helped him find the answer he needed.

There have been several studies into the effects of walking in nature. The best known was conducted by Marc Berman, Assistant Professor of Psychology and Cognitive Neuroscience at The University of Chicago, who investigated whether walking in nature can improve our ability to concentrate and pay attention. He sent groups of students out to walk, first in a park in the city of Ann Arbor, Michigan, then the following week in busy urban streets nearby. Their mood, levels of attention, and other measures were rigorously tested before and after each process. Berman then repeated the experiment, this time using photographs of scenery in Nova Scotia and North American urban spaces. He found clear evidence that cognitive performance was much improved in the group who encountered nature either physically or via photographs.[xxiii]

Gregory Bratman, a conservation biologist at Stanford University, conducted a similar study. He assigned sixty participants to a 50-minute walk in either a natural or an urban environment in and around Stanford, California, and ran a series of psychological assessments before and after the walk. The nature walk resulted in measurably decreased anxiety and rumination as well as improvements in memory, but the results from the urban walk were significantly lower. He repeated the experiment with the addition of before-and-after brain scans, and got the same kinds of results.[xxiv]

Of course, these experiments only serve to support what we've known for millennia. As Thoreau once observed 'Methinks that the moment my legs begin to move, my thoughts begin to flow.[xxv]

Mucking out the burros

Carolyn Miller is a screenwriter with a long career of writing for Hollywood movies and TV shows. She is also a pioneering digital storyteller and author of the very successful 'Digital Storytelling, a Creator's Guide to Interactive Entertainment'. Her portfolio includes an early interactive version of *Toy Story* and the video game *Where in the World is Carmen Sandiego*? Most recently, she was on the narrative team for an immersive story-based world: *Meow Wolf's House of Eternal Return.*

Born in San Francisco, she lived in Los Angeles for many years but in 2012 she and her husband bought a house and some land in Santa Fe where she has finally been able to realise a lifelong dream – to own a pair of burros (or donkeys, as they are known in the UK).

I interviewed Carolyn to find out how she was managing to integrate a very online life with raising and training burros. This is what she told me:

'I have a very close relationship with the digital world, in part because my living depends on it, and in part because it's my major form of communication. I'm online constantly, via my laptop computer, from the time I get up to the time I go to bed. Even if I'm not sitting in front of it, it's on and I catch up on news and emails whenever I pass by my office. I also really like my iPad, and it's loaded with apps. I have an iPhone but since we live out in the country, it gets terrible reception so I often forget to check my messages on it.

'In terms of social media, I use Facebook, Twitter and LinkedIn. I find LinkedIn the most valuable professionally and have had some excellent opportunities come from LinkedIn messages I got out of the blue. As for synergies between working in digital media and owning burros, I do see some, primarily in the balance it gives to my life. Before I became a burro owner, I would sit in front of my laptop virtually all day, writing or doing research. My neck and back often ached and I know I was often on the grumpy side.

'But once I acquired the donkeys, I've had no choice but to go outside to feed and water them and to muck out the barn. I admit there have been days when I didn't feel like going out, especially in bad weather, but I've always been happy once I stepped out the door. Taking care of them, and getting out in the fresh air this way has been a great way to clear my head and get re-energized. I think overall I'm more cheerful than I used to be and my back and neck feel better. Also, as I go about the routine of caring for them, I've come up with some great ideas for my book and for other work I'm doing, just out of the blue. And oddly enough, I've found raking up the manure to be a highly satisfying job. It's physical work, so I consider it my "gym," and it feels very good to clean up the barn and haul away a big wheel barrow of manure, and to leave everything neat and tidy. A little side note here: I was amazed at how much manure two donkeys could produce, especially since they are much smaller than horses!'.

I asked whether she saw her technological concerns as very different from her 'real life'. She said

'My technological concerns *are* my real life! I'm far too involved with digital media to make any separation. And I get panicky when things go wrong with technology, so I don't think I'm a very good geek. Last night, for instance, as I was working on a document, my cursor started to twitch and vibrate and I wasn't able to stop it. I couldn't save what I was working on and I couldn't continue to write. In the end, I had to reboot, which made me lose everything new that I had written since my last save. It was extremely frustrating. My donkeys couldn't help me there!'

I wondered whether she thinks it's good for geeky people to get outdoors and interact with animals?

'It has definitely been beneficial in my case, though a much larger commitment of time than I had anticipated. It has also made my life a lot more complicated, with many new concerns. I now have to worry about the price of hay and where I will get the hay from and about my hay getting mouldy when it rains or snows. I also have to make sure my burros are in good health, which means I have to arrange for regular visits from the farrier and the vet. I've particularly enjoyed my interactions with my two "girls" and observing their very different personalities. It has made my life much richer than it was before and they have given me some good laughs.' Now, she and her burro Pearl are both in training – Pearl to pull a buggy and Carolyn to drive her.

As far as technology is concerned, she thinks we should spend more time on the positives.

'What about 'technological blessings?' At present, I see new advances in technology as giving us new ways to tell stories, and I find that very exciting. But at times, I do feel overwhelmed with the continual flow of technological advances, and struggle to keep current. Sometimes I would just like to yell "STOP!" to give us time to fully explore what we already have.'

Carolyn Miller has found that the demanding physical work of taking care of burros has brought more balance to her daily wired life. And it's not just the routine labour that's satisfying, but also the regular contact with the donkeys themselves

E.O. Wilson says that 'we are human in good part because of the particular way we affiliate with other organisms'.[xxvi] Philosopher Paul Shepard believes that images of animals in early cave art, such as the astounding drawings found in caves in Chauvet, France, and thought to be over 30,000 years old, could have helped to internalize key images shared by a group. They may, he thinks, characterize 'a root of biophilia, that's in us still, the tug of attention to animals as the curved mirror of ourselves'. [xxvii]

For Carolyn, this tug of attention is answered in the hard and intimate work of looking after living animals. For others, the mirror may be found in simple interior decoration. Animals are already understood to be a significant element of the biophilic environment. According to social ecologist Stephen Kellert, the presence of animal forms in design often provokes satisfaction, pleasure, stimulation and emotional interest, and they are frequently represented in building interiors 'through the use of ornament, decoration, art, and in stylized and highly metaphorical disguise'.[xxviii]

Organic materials bridge the gap

I once posted on Twitter about the benefits of wooden computer kit, and promptly received the following intriguing reply from a user by the name of @backwards7: 'I'd like to own a mouse made from organic materials that would gradually wear away to the shape of my hand.'

More information followed via direct message:

'The leather strap of one of my old watches has distinctive kinks in it which were sculpted by my wrist. I've personalised it, not by saying 'This is mine' but rather through my continuous interaction with it. One of the problems with technology is that it's designed to be disposable and immutable. I've made no impression on the plastic strap of my Fitbit. Externally, my iPod Nano, which is on the desk in front of me as I write this, looks the same as it did when I bought it in 2008.'

Effective haptic technologies are something of a Holy Grail in interface design. Haptics is the science of applying touch, or tactile, sensations to interaction with computer applications. The word comes from a Greek root meaning 'to fasten', and is an important pathway between the world of abstract data and the physical universe. If you have ever held a video game controller in your hands, for example, you have probably felt it vibrate when it performs certain actions. It seems to 'fasten' your connection between the virtual and the real.

Haptics science is still in its infancy but there's no

reason not to create, or be aware of, your own touch pathways, as happened with @backwards7 in the case of the leather strap.

I'm also reminded of the writer Roger Deakin, a nature geek rather than a techie geek, who hollowed out a space in the surface of his desk until it was just the right size to contain a smooth pebble he had collected in the Hebrides. It was, he said, 'like a tiny curling stone, a sort of worry-bead.'

I love this idea. Even just the simple act of sanding down the hollow could provide a deeply ritualistic moment in an otherwise digital day. My own wooden desk has no hollows yet, but I'm working on it. Once it a while, I get a ritualistic pleasure from clearing away the papers, cables, and computer, and applying a new layer of polish to its surface. Just because digital activities take place on it, doesn't mean it can't be enjoyed as an organic entity in its own right.

Stephen Kellert was inspired by E.O. Wilson's work on biophilia to champion a new architectural practice he called *biophilic design*, connecting buildings to the natural world in order to create environments where people feel and perform better. Designs might include gardens, water features, and shapes mimicking those from nature like shells and foliage. They would feature natural materials, plenty of light, and open spaces. The aim is to repair environmental damage and restore sustainability by paying attention to beneficial contact between people and nature in modern buildings and landscapes.

Technobiophilic design is a natural extension of this concept. Recently, technobiophilic notions have begun to appear in the toolboxes of designers, planners and architects around the world. Just as we still desire homes to live in, so we also want access to positive and rewarding technologies. To paraphrase Stephen Kellert, technobiophilic design connects our digital lives to the natural world so we can feel and perform better.

Tim Beatley, Teresa Heinz Professor of

Sustainable Communities at the University of Virginia, looks forward to 'the promise and potential of technobiophilic cities, that at once commit to restoring and enjoying actual nature, but acknowledge the realities of life in cities (much of it inside, and behind a screen), and the powerful ways in which our digital technologies could underpin and help to reinforce our natureful commitments and experiences and our biophilic tendencies'.[xxix]

Being away

Novelist Sarah Boxer wrote this gorgeous description of reading on your mobile in bed:

'Your cellphone screen is like a tiny glass-bottomed boat moving slowly over a vast and glowing ocean of words in the night. There is no shore. There is nothing beyond the words in front of you. It is a voyage for one in the night-time. Pure romance'.[xxx]

She allowed herself to be transported, not just by

the contents of her reading, but also by the delightful physicality of her mobile phone.

Then there's the story of a leukaemia patient in Dorset County Hospital in England. She is confined to an isolation ward where the windows are kept tightly shut and her exposure to airborne bacteria is carefully monitored. Normally there wouldn't be much to see through the windows from her bed but each morning, after a painful and sleepless night, she lies in her bed and watches the sun come up over the sea. Even though Poole Bay is several miles away, she can follow every moment of the growing light as it glitters on the incoming tide and highlights the tips of pine trees in a dawn shower of pink streaks and scattered clouds.

She is watching a live video stream provided by the charity Arts in Hospital. It's part of a pioneering arts project called Room With a View, designed especially for patients whose treatment involves periods of isolation. A live feed is projected from two locations: a camera on the roof of Kingston Maurward House, approximately three kilometres away, showing the gardens and the lake, and a seascape captured from the roof of Brownsea Castle. The images are transmitted to large LCD screens in two isolation rooms used for immuno-compromised patients with leukaemia and other blood cancers. Now, during those long terrible nights when a seriously ill patient lies awake in pain, or is afraid and can't sleep, they can at least watch the passages of the sun and moon.

The Kaplans consolidated their extensive research in the development of Attention Restoration Theory. ART, as it has come to be called, features a number of situations, or 'settings', each of which provides a different kind of experience. One of these is called 'being away', and it could be applied to watching nature on a screen. Live or static, it comes into play when you find yourself in a place or state of mind that's physically or conceptually different from your usual environment.

It works, they say, because we experience the

world conceptually as well as physically, so the experience of being away involves what's going on in your head just as much as your physical environment. The Kaplans use the example of stepping outside for a moment: 'Even if you travel no further than your own garden,' they wrote, 'making the rounds to find new buds and make sure all is well can feel like being quite distant from the world of pressures and obligations'.

The same applies whether you're moved by the glowing rectangle of e-book in the dark or a virtual sunrise projected through the internet just for you.

Thinking of getting a digital detox?

Now that we're all connected, the new status symbol has become the wherewithal to live offline, according to journalist Gaby Hinsliff.[xxxi] And what better way to try it out than by taking a digital detox?

The idea is simple. Health detoxes are already fashionable – you spend a few days once or twice a year cleansing your system of various toxic substances which are believed to build up in the body as a result of our stressed-out junk food lifestyle.

A digital detox works on a similar principle, except that you abstain not from rich food, cigarettes and alcohol, but from your electronics. A period spent away from email is thought to cleanse your brain of nasty social media habits and restore clarity and mental wellbeing. It is, says Hinsliff, 'a bit like colonic irrigation for the mind, flushing out all the unnecessary gunge'.

It can be quite simply achieved by disconnecting yourself from the internet and turning off your phone for short bursts of time This will, it is hoped, flush out the anxiety infesting your poor wired mind. Benefits of switching off are said to include reduced stress, an increased sense of calm, better sleep and a sense of freedom, although to date I've been unable to find a respectable research project which supports those claims.

Numerous studies and anecdotal reports have

shown that being out in nature can be very restorative. But does turning off your kit increase the benefit? And is it worth the bother and expense?

Some hardliners go offline for a whole year, but usually only to write a book about it. Or you might purchase a detox vacation in some area of wild natural beauty where others take control of your consumption by confiscating your kit and enticing you towards other kinds of social and unwired interactions.

Under the banner 'Disconnect to Reconnect', for example, the US-based Camp Grounded invites you to 'trade in your computer, cell phone, email, Instagrams, clocks, schedules, work-jargon, networking events and conferences for an off-the-grid weekend of pure unadulterated fun in the redwoods', 'celebrating what it means to be alive'.

Or try the Caribbean island of St Vincent and the Grenadines, where a digital detox holiday package lets travellers exchange their smartphones for a guidebook explaining how to function without technology and also provides a life coach to help them through it.

There's no harm in taking a holiday away from the internet, of course, but an increasing number of people are finding that actually staying offline permanently is not an option. Your job may demand that you're contactable via email or, if you don't have a job, it could be the Government that's insisting you manage your benefits online. Then there's banking, buying and selling, booking travel, and of course socialising, plus a million other reasons to log on.

Sociologist Nathan Jurgenson argues that 'unplugging' from the internet is not about restoring the self so much as it is about stifling the desire for autonomy that technology can inspire.'[xxxii] The fantasy, he suggests, is to cast off the virtual and re-embrace the tangible through disconnecting and undertaking a purifying digital detox in which 'one can reconnect with the real, the meaningful – one's true self that rejects social media's seductive velvet cage'.

So are we kidding ourselves that handing in our phones at the door and spending a weekend gambolling in a forest will free us from the thrall of technology? Perhaps.

I would like to propose another kind of resort, one which offers not detoxification but intoxication – with nature *and* digital life. The ingredients are an outstandingly beautiful forest, beach or wilderness with a comfortable hostelry in your preferred style, lots of pleasurable group and solo activities, and lashings of wifi. You can gaze at the stars each night while tracking the International Space Station on your iPad; take wonderful photos and share them on Facebook, and journal the entire experience on whatever platform you like best.

Turn messages and GPS on or off, as is your pleasure.

And remember - if you have all that kit in the first place, you're a lucky grown-up living in the 21st century: enjoy it.[xxxiii]

Loving FarmVille

Do you harvest tomatoes in FarmVille in your lunch break? If so, you're probably reaping some biophilic benefits from digital nearby nature.

FarmVille, for those unfamiliar with it, is an online game accessed through Facebook. It provides a nostalgic homestead in the countryside and the chance to create, build and nourish the farm of your dreams. Players cultivate their own land, ploughing, planting and harvesting crops. They also care for their farm animals, milking cows and collecting eggs from their own chickens.

The game has attracted some interesting collaborations, most notably with Cascadian Farm, a real-life organic foods company. On its website, Cascadian extols the sumptuous virtues of its Home Farm, 'nestled in the foothills of the breath-taking North Cascades mountain range' where you can stop at roadside stands to buy a pint of berries or homemade organic ice cream.

In 2010, Cascadian Farm stepped into the online

world when it ran a month-long promotion in the online FarmVille Market. Its aim was to sell a crop of 310 million virtual organic blueberries. Within a week, over a million players had bought non-existent packs of non-existent blueberries at a cost of 20 FarmVille credits each (around US $4), according to Mashable.[xxxiv]

Zynga, the company behind FarmVille, got in touch when Slate published my piece 'Gazing at Virtual Nature Is Good for Your Psychological Well-Being'.[xxxv] Apparently, my research matched up with their own findings from extensive focus group testing into the reasons why people play the game, but they had not heard of biophilia nor seen the environmental psychology studies which explained those reasons. They told me that a fair percentage of players reported feeling strongly connected to nature when they played FarmVille, and many used it to relax and de-stress. Some players who had no access to their own piece of land saw it as a substitute for real gardening.

Their experience correlates with those described by Holly Nielsen in an interesting Guardian article on what she calls 'sentimental pastoralism' in video games.[xxxvi] She writes 'there has been a discovery that the uncertainties and rhythms of farming make good gaming fodder. Zynga's early Facebook game FarmVille was a spectacular success, attracting over 40 million active users, with its simplified take on crop production and animal care'. There are other farming games, too, such as 'Farming Simulator' which, she says, 'has shown that there's a mass audience for authentic simulation complete with branded machinery and multiple authentic livestock breeds'.

Nielsen admits she's not immune to the seduction of the idealised rural life. 'Throughout history humans have been preoccupied with understanding and 'getting back' to a Golden Age of natural harmony – which of course never really existed. In our efforts to associate with this 'purer' existence, we've idealised the experience of rural life. Video games are just the latest means of doing that. Since moving to London I've found myself craving titles such as Animal Crossing and Story of Seasons. Like Marie Antoinette playing at being a milkmaid in her purpose built farm, I delve into an equally superficial homestead to sate my desire for simplicity and escape.'

The benefits of FarmVille and the many other games discussed in Nielsen's article are not just biophilic; they offer a sense of a nature-based community too, one which is subject to the seasons, the passage of the sun, and the shared day-to-day earthiness of country toil. Together, the players come together to raise barns, collect in crops, and rescue each other from natural calamities.

In real life it's easy to see how, when sitting at your office desk, squeezed into a corner on a busy commuter train, or relaxing at the end of a day of abstract and apparently meaningless work, you can enjoy tending your virtual garden and caring for your online cows and sheep.

The landscapes of Grand Theft Auto

It's so frustrating. I've been driving round the city for over an hour trying to find the freeway that will get me out of here and up into the mountains. The streets are jangling with the noise of squealing brakes and revving engines. People on the sidewalks yell at each other and step into the road without looking; I'm constantly having to swerve to avoid them. Where the hell is that freeway entrance? I consult the spread of paper wobbling across my knees. I'm feeling nauseous from looking down at the map then up ahead and steering at the same time. I can see it's close but I just can't find the ramp. Then, all of a sudden, I'm on it. Not sure how that happened but I'm on the freeway and, I hope, going east. From there the plan is to find a dirt track to take me into Blaine County with its beautiful empty wilderness. Peace and quiet, eagles, sloping fields of scented flowers… that's what I'm hoping for. But right now I need to focus on keeping the vehicle on the road.

Suddenly, I press the wrong button and - BAM - the screen fades momentarily. When it returns I'm back in the Clifton Avenue car park where I started. Dammit. It took me this long to find a route out and finally get on the freeway but now my mistake has hurled me back to the start of the game.

I'm learning to play Grand Theft Auto V and it's not going well. Why, you might ask, do I even care about it? I'm not a gamer, and the violent sexist world of GTA with its cursing, robbery and murder certainly doesn't appeal to me. Except, that is, for one small thing: I've heard that the landscapes in GTA V are breathtakingly beautiful. In fact, they are so good there's even a Flickr photo-sharing group dedicated to their appreciation.

I first heard about the community of 'Landscape photographers of Los Santos and Blaine County' in 2014. It was created by photographer Phil Rose as a place for members to share pictures taken inside the game. Many of the photos are glorious in their detail, although their smooth patina of graphic design acts as a reminder that these landscapes

84

are grown from pixels rather than soil. But the vantage points from which they are taken can feel as if the photographer was physically there next to this tree or beneath that sky. There are beaches, lakes, meadows, and towering mountains, all based on the wildlands of Southern California.

I should explain that California is the country of my heart. I've visited many times and lived there for a short while. The first time I saw the Flickr photos I was instantly reminded me of the day I visited the Santa Ynez Mountains just above Santa Barbara. I had been invited to join some friends on a trip up to the high slopes. It was springtime, when they burst into bloom and attract a steady flow of admirers. Since I was a foreigner, I knew nothing of this phenomenon, and anyway I usually preferred to turn my gaze westwards towards the Pacific. The mountains to the east formed a dark forbidding background I seldom thought about. But that day, I saw astonishing drifts of red, yellow, purple, and blue flowing across the rocky contours like an ocean of tiny petals. The scene was unforgettable.

So it was that, years later, the Flickr pictures brought back powerful memories of that magical day in the mountains and, along with them, a burning longing to return. At that time, I wasn't in a position to travel halfway across the world to experience that landscape once again, but perhaps I could visit in virtual life. Perhaps, via the game, I could explore the high chaparrals once more. And that's what got me started in GTA V.

Grand Theft Auto is set in the fictional city of San Andreas and its surrounds, but its features blatantly bear more than a passing resemblance to Los Angeles and Southern California. You can drive out from the city and through the suburbs to reach beaches, lakes, meadows, and towering mountains, all eerily based on the real thing.

I started my gaming life with high hopes. Soon, I thought, I would be wandering the slopes and enjoying the peace and quiet. Wrong. I had assumed I could just log in and somehow teleport to my destination, just as you do in Second Life. But no. The game is way too rule-based for that. I would have to travel to the mountains by road, and in order to finance the trip I would have to steal, kill and drive my way out of the city. Maybe I would be lucky enough to hijack a helicopter and get out faster, but first it would help if I could actually keep the car on the road.

So, back to the present. Perched on a stool in front of the TV with the PS3 console in my hands, I consult the map on my knee, press R3 to accelerate, then thumb L1 to steer my way out of the carpark and back onto the road. Dusk is falling fast in San Andreas but the darkening peaks are still just visible in the distance as I head towards them once more.

As we saw earlier, Marc Berman found that walking round a park produced more beneficial effects than walking in an urban environment. Psychologist Deltcho Valtchanov wanted to find out if the same test would work in a virtual reality. He set up a variation of Berman's experiment using not real parks and streets, but three VR spaces: a nature island with waterfalls, rivers, different kinds of trees, flowers, plants, grass, rocks, a beach and dirt paths; an assortment of 3D geometric shapes including coloured spheres, cylinders, cones, and rectangular and square boxes of various sizes; and a scale model of Shibuya station in Tokyo, a dense urban area with realistic and full-scale buildings and streets which was unfamiliar to any participants. [xxxvii]

Using Berman's methods, he tested the reactions of 69 subjects and found that the virtual nature space prompted an increase in positive affect – happiness, friendliness, affection and playfulness. At the same time negative affect – fear, anger and sadness – decreased. Results in the other two spaces, the geometric shapes and Shibuya station, were far less marked. Valtchanov had originally wondered whether the simple state of being in VR might trigger positive benefits, but this experiment convinced him otherwise. It was definitely a combination of VR plus nature that caused them.

It seems possible that, in some instances at least,

digital experience could perhaps replace analogue with no reduction in benefit. Consider, for example, the outcome of a Spanish advertising campaign which showed, in a rather worrying way, that simulated nature experiences can be remarkably powerful.

In a 2008 study of Spanish energy consumers,[xxxviii] researchers Hartmann and Apaolaza-Ibáñez examined responses to a new marketing idea from one of the leading energy brands, Iberdrola Energia Verde. The company was trying to green up its image with a TV campaign that would evoke virtual nature experiences by way of pleasant nature imagery such as flying eagles, mountain scenery, and waterfalls.

Consumers responded quickly and very positively to the new branding. Analysts found that of the broad group of people in their sample, from those who were already environmentally conscious to others with much less interest, all experienced 'warm glow' benefits and a positive feeling of contributing to the common good. These results worried the researchers. 'Because our society has become more urbanized and it is increasingly difficult for people to get access to nature', they wrote, 'people will tend to experience simulated nature experiences through their exposure to virtual nature in the media'. What concerned them was that it seemed their sample of users experienced just the same positives as if they had encountered real nature. Virtual nature was indeed meeting their human desires to experience nature, and awarding them the same psychological benefits.

If the effect of virtual nature is as powerful as they found it to be in that one example, future urban populations in dense cities with very little natural greenery could be subjected to surrogate 'calming' experiences without ever having access to living nature. A frightening and depressing prospect.

Where am I?

In 1995, Nicholas Negroponte wrote: 'Digital living will include less and less dependence upon being in a specific place at a specific time, and the transmission of place itself will start to become possible. If I could really look out the electronic window of my living room in Boston and see the Alps, hear the cowbells, and smell the (digital) manure in summer, in a way I'm very much in Switzerland'.[xxxix]*

As founder of the MIT Media Lab, and an architect by trade, he knew what he was talking about twenty plus years ago. It's taken quite a while to even begin to make his vision a reality, but we're getting closer.

I was reminded of it when I learned that, in recent years, several cruise companies have installed virtual balconies on their ships. The cheapest accommodation on ocean-going liners has always been the windowless inside cabin, but now many of them sport an 80-inch high-definition screen showing a live real-time feed of the ocean outside. High-speed cameras placed strategically around the ship ensure that the feeds match the placing of the cabins and show the view passengers would have, if only their cabin wall was on the outside of the ship.

Other ships offer virtual balconies. They look just like a real balcony, complete with curtains, but nothing is real. 'Even when you are right up next to it, it looks like you could reach straight through it,' according to Bill Martin, Chief Information Officer at Royal Caribbean.[xl] The installation even includes live sound which matches what you would hear if you were sitting on a real balcony.

In 2011, the Disney Cruise Line tried circular 'virtual portholes' but haven't installed them in their newer ships, purportedly because of the cost, but perhaps because a simulated porthole is less satisfying to our biophilic needs than a simulated balcony.

Such features are good examples of the Kaplans'

concept of 'extent'. Extent involves being in a setting which is so rich and coherent that it engages the mind and promotes exploration. In Japanese bonsai gardens, the miniature trees, rocks and gravel create extent through intensity rather than through the suggestion of distance. An entire world, a complete microcosm, can be captured in a tiny space. Or, perhaps, in a digital facsimile.

Another example of extent can be found in an app called Flyover Country.[xli] It was developed at the University of Minnesota with funding from the National Science Foundation, and is designed to be used in aircraft. How often have you sat on a plane staring out of the window at the most amazing landscapes with absolutely no idea of where they are or even which country you're flying over? Now you can learn about the world along the path of your flight. The app analyses your route and caches geologic maps and interactive points of interest. It can then display the locations of fossils and georeferenced Wikipedia articles about the landscapes 3,000 feet below.

Airline companies and tourist destinations have also taken up the idea of a virtual view and developed VR trailers to market their wares. Some packages include panoramic videos that can be viewed online, via YouTube and Facebook, whilst others require apps and special viewers like Oculus Rift or Google Cardboard. The idea is that trying out a location virtually can help holiday-makers get a more immersive sense of the place, after which they will want to go there for real.

Potential destinations range from Connecticut's Mohegan Sun casino and entertainment resort, to Las Vegas, British Columbia and the South Pacific archipelago of New Caledonia, all of which offer VR experiences they hope will transform viewers into visitors.

But why bother to travel physically at all? You can already take virtual reality trips to a growing list of exotic locations such as Nepal, for example, where you can join The North Face climber and filmmaker Renan Ozturk on his Spring 2015 adventure; or

Machu Picchu, Rwanda, Iceland, or the Arctic – they can all be explored in VR.

I wonder if it's possible to take a virtual reality trip to a digital detox camp? That would be a head-spinner.

The joy of surfing

In 1992, internet enthusiast Jean Armour Polly was commissioned to write an article introducing the net to her fellow librarians. By then it was already more than 20 years old, but few people had heard of it or knew how to use it. When she began writing, she wanted to describe to her readers how it feels to go online.

'I needed something that would evoke a sense of randomness, chaos, and even danger. I wanted something fishy, net-like, nautical', she wrote later.

As she cast around for the right metaphor, her glance fell on her mousepad. There, beneath her hand, was a picture of a surfer. The pad was a gift to her from its designer, Steve Cisler, who was based at Apple HQ in Cupertino, California. For Polly, a land-locked librarian in Syracuse, New York, with no connections to surf culture and not even a keen swimmer, it made perfect sense.

'Eureka', she said later, 'I had my metaphor'. She called the article 'Surfing the Internet'. It appeared in the Wilson Library Bulletin in 1992 and marked the first published use of the term.

Since then the notion of surfing the internet has been picked up worldwide by people who have never mounted a board, perhaps never even seen a beach, yet their imaginations are fired by the idea of carefree riding in a sea of information.

'Water makes you happier, more connected and better at what you do', says Wallace J Nichols, a marine biologist and wild water advocate based at the California Academy of Sciences in San Francisco. In his book 'Blue Mind'[xlii], Nichols explains the benefits of simply looking at images of seas, lakes and rivers.

He describes an experiment at Plymouth University in 2010 when 40 adults were asked to rate pictures of different natural and urban environments. The researchers found that any picture containing water triggered higher ratings for positive mood, preference and perceived restorativeness, than those images with no water, no matter whether they were shown in a natural landscape or an urban setting. Other experiments have supported these findings.

We're used to associating the colour green with environmental wellbeing, but less attention has been paid to 'blue' areas such as beaches, lakes, rivers and the ocean. However, studies of the impact of blue space on human health and wellbeing are growing in number. The concept of Blue Mind, Nichols says, is about the 'human-ocean connection', an emotional bond whose roots may in the future be charted by neuroscientists.

This kind of research is attracting marine biologists, conservationists, artists, urban planners – indeed, anyone interested in the relationship between humanity and our watery planet. The interdisciplinary Blue Gym project at the University of Exeter Medical School has been investigating the psychological and physical health benefits of exposure to natural water environments. They have found that the stress levels of people living in coastal communities may be lower than normal simply because they spend more of their leisure time near, or even in, the sea.[xliii]

When I was researching 'Technobiophilia' I found that surfing is not the only example of watery metaphors to be found in cyberspace. We swim in our Twitter streams, dive into torrent files, float on data clouds. All kinds of waterfalls, babbling brooks, and ubiquitous ocean views can be found on desktops and home screens around the world. 'This wallpaper brings the sunny beach to you,' says the blurb for Beach Live Wallpaper. 'The waves in summer time break on the shore right on your phone.' The blue mind can be right inside your digital life.

Experimenting with virtual reality

Virtual reality is still in its infancy but design studios are already testing ambitious VR experiences in Oculus Rift, Samsung Gear and other systems. If you have a headset, you can take a cinematic virtual reality observational journey following the lives of nomadic yak herders in Mongolia. Or how about an Oculus Rift planetarium in your living room, complete with an astronomer to show you around? If you're a fan of Second Life you'll soon be able to explore Project Sansar, a new world designed especially for VR where users can create their own experiences and visit other people's. If the original Second Life is anything to go by, there will be many colourful new landscapes to investigate.

If you don't yet have access to that level of technology, try the very inexpensive Google Cardboard. You'll be astonished to discover that you can get an incredible virtual reality experience using just a simple cardboard box. Google

Cardboard has been championed by The New York Times, which even gave one away to all its readers. The NYTVR app gives you the chance to walk through a herd of powerful American Bison, some of whom seem to come right up and peer into your face. You can almost smell their breath. Recently, I happened to be cuddled up on the sofa looking at books with my small grandson when he pointed to a picture of bison roaming the plains and said he wondered what it would be like to be really close up to them. (He is a boy of many questions.)

Well, I was able to reply, delighted to get the chance to segue from print to digital, let us try this! I got out my Google Cardboard, which he had already played with several times, and ran the NYTVR bison. He twisted this way and that as he moved between the great creatures. Beyond the headset, I could hear their heavy snorts and dusty hooves on the ground. There was no odour, of course, no body heat, no real sense of dangerous proximity, and yet it was intense. I suppose you would call it a different kind of real.

That day I glimpsed the future of education. He was only three years old, unable yet to read or write, but he had already learned how to 'read' virtual reality in an intuitive way. And this is how he will probably be learning on a regular basis throughout his schooldays and beyond. What kind of contact with virtual nature will he have when he is ten? Fifteen? I can't begin to imagine, but I expect it will involve not just sound and vision, but also smell, touch, probably even taste. You can already get immersive nasal simulators which generate the aromas of virtual food, flowers, perfumes, and other things you would maybe rather not smell. The menu to date includes hay grass, flowers, ocean, jungle, rain, fields and strawberries (remember that ancient biophilic memory?) all at $4.99 each.[xliv]

The mission of Oculus Rift is to 'make it possible to experience anything, anywhere'. Make no mistake, VR is poised to change the way we encounter the natural world, and the only way to understand how is to engage with it in a conscious and mindful way. It's only when we have experience of it that we will begin to understand what we're dealing with, what nature could become in the technobiophilic future, and which options might be open to us.

Jeremy Bailenson directs The Virtual Human Interaction Lab at Stanford University. His team try to understand the ways in which people react to VR and how it can be used to improve empathy, conservation and communications. Their research has demonstrated that if you show somebody the consequences of their actions in virtual reality it can make them rethink their behaviour in the real world. 'With concepts like climate change, deforestation, or pollution, we can use virtual reality to make the relationship between human behaviour and the impact on the environment less abstract and more concrete'.[xlv]

Virtual reality does three things, explains Bailenson. First, it tracks your physical movements in the world; then it uses that data to redraw a scene, and finally it sends out new perceptual information to the eyes, ears and skin so that you perceive the effect of your actions and respond accordingly.

But there's a paradox, he says, in that although it feels like reality, it's far from it. 'The brain treats the experience as real, but we can create any experience fathomable.' This, of course, is the 'virtual' in virtual reality. This can be rewarding, but also very confusing and, of course, alarming. We're going to need a whole new kind of literacy to understand what's happening.

Take, for example, Bailenson's 'Fish Avatars' research project. It gathers data about the real movement of electronically tagged fish in the kelp forests of Monterey Bay, then uses it to programme a VR environment where humans can enter the virtual underwater realm and observe virtual versions of live fish. Researchers then gather data in turn from the human participants about the way they relate to the virtual avatars of the real fish. The purpose of the research is, by the way, to study the

103

behaviour of the people, not the fish.

When Facebook acquired Oculus Rift for two billion dollars, Mark Zuckerberg wrote 'By feeling truly present, you can share unbounded spaces and experiences with the people in your life. Imagine sharing not just moments with your friends online, but entire experiences and adventures.'[xlvi]

What kinds of adventures? We watch and wait. But one thing is for sure – just like those unwary fish in the kelp forest, our data will be harvested every step of the way.

CyberParks

Visit an urban park on a sunny day and you'll see people relaxing with newspapers, books and, of course, phones and tablets. The digital has become part of our outdoor lives and the trend is set to continue.

If you have been to Paris recently, you may have come across a curious installation at the busy Rond Point des Champs-Elysées. 'Escale Numérique' (translated as Digital Break) was designed by Mathieu Lehanneur. He got his inspiration from the city's 19th-century network of drinking fountains, but this time he tapped not into an underground water source, but a fibre optic network, creating a fountain of free wifi. The structure has a large touch screen protected by a sustainable green roof covered with plants, and concrete swivel seats with mini tables and electric points. It offers a tantalising glimpse into how urban tech/nature balance might look in the new few years' time.

Travel to The Netherlands, and you may see Daan Roosegaarde's glowing Van Gogh cycle path. It's a kilometre-long segment of cycle route through the Dutch province of Noord Brabant, where the artist was born and raised. The illuminated swirling patterns echo his night-time paintings. The specially-coated surface is power by a solar panel and, on cloudy days, LEDs along the side of the path cast extra light where needed.

And in Poland, the Botanical Garden of Adam Mickiewicz University in Poznan features geolocated trees and an ornithological educational path designed to inform users about nearby bird life. The path has its own app, information panels, and QR codes which activate recordings of birdsong. The mission here leans towards education rather than wellbeing or art, but each has its place in the new ecosystem of cyberparks.

I'm a member of the CyberParks network, a large European research group established to find ways of using new technologies to encourage more people to spend time outside. In the past, the natural environment and the digital domain were seen as distinctly different, miles apart both physically and culturally. But the growth of social media, wearable tech such as smartwatches, mobile connectivity, plus the fact that we now carry the internet in our pockets, is profoundly influencing the way we experience time, space, and other people. The transdisciplinary CyberParks team of urban planners, anthropologists, architects, artists, engineers, computer scientists, geographers, interaction designers and psychologists comes together to plan the near-future. They see a park as an intelligent environment where the landscape itself responds to people moving through it, and where sensors and computers are seamlessly embedded to enhance the traditional park activities we treasure. And they all agree on one thing – that however digital it might get, the essence of the park is still all about being outdoors and experiencing nature.

There's increasing interest from public policy makers in the amount of time we spend outdoors. In 2009, Natural England commissioned the Monitor of Engagement with the Natural Environment survey[xlvii]. Its brief was to find out how we, the public, use and enjoy the outdoors. The team found that while 54% of the adult population normally visited open spaces in and around towns and cities, such as parks, canals and nature areas, coasts and beaches; or countryside areas such as farm and woodland, hills and rivers at least once a week, a further 10% of respondents reported they had not visited the great outdoors in the previous twelve months, while 8% had made only one or two visits.

Yet, there's evidence that people do seek to spend time in green spaces, even if they are bite-sized and squeezed into the working day. In a report for environmental consultants Terrapin Bright Green, Sam Gochman writes 'If you choose to take your lunch break outside rather than sitting at your desk, chances are you prefer a place that has nature or natural elements (pocket park, grassy lawn, views to water, etc). Biophilia, our innate connection with nature, subconsciously steers us to places that allow us to experience nature and natural elements.'[xlviii] The company surveyed 100 people on their lunch breaks at four sites—two biophilic and two non-biophilic—in lower Manhattan. They found that a large proportion of participants at biophilic sites liked at least one natural or 'biophilic' element most about those spaces and cited both convenience and access to nature as the most important factors in choosing those spaces. Most said that they would be willing to walk a longer distance to get to a space with more nature.

Make something technobiophilic

Technobiophilic design connects our digital lives to the natural world so we can feel and perform better. Just as architects design houses with turf roofs, and interior designers create water features and green walls inside buildings, we should be applying the principles of technobiophilia to the hardware and software we make. Why is there so much plastic and metal in digital culture? What about wood and other natural fabrics? Why so many straight lines? Why not curves and circles?

I've been hoping that someone would come up with a technobiophilia app or, even better, a wearable. Something that clearly demonstrates the levels of wellbeing to be gained from a technobiophilic lifestyle. How about applying technobiophilic design to software and hardware? More natural materials and colours please!

There are many apps which measure heart rate, blood pressure, and other body functions. But is there a way to collect and cross-reference that data with information about the environment they are in?

A technobiophilic tracker could measure how my heart rate changes when I go from my office to sitting in a green park, walking in a forest or relaxing on the beach. It could watch and analyse physical and locational parameters to generate a scale of my wellbeing and track it over time, and allow me to share and compare the results. It could help me learn how to develop less stressful behaviours. As far as I know there are, as yet, no apps which do anything like this.

That's the challenge I offer to designers and developers. Please, make something technobiophilic for me!

The closest I've come to it was in 2014 when I was asked to speak at Sesi Cultura Digital in Rio de Janeiro. It was a large hackathon, where teams of programmers and designers work together to invent and create new computer applications. Unfortunately I was unable to take up their fantastic offer and travel to Brazil at that time, so instead the organisers invited me to create a technobiophilic challenge for participants to work on. Could they devise some software or hardware that connected nature with technology to promote wired wellbeing?

One group of designers from the Nucleus of Art and New Organisms, a transdisciplinary hothouse of artistic and engineering talent in Rio de Janeiro, came up with Symbio, a very clever project which won second prize. They had already worked with plants, bees, sound and the body, so when they read about the concept of technobiophilia they immediately saw its relevance. They decided to create a technological bridge between people and nature.

The idea behind Symbio is simple: if you lead a healthy life, your houseplant will thrive. If you don't, it withers and dies.

It's made up of a wearable device, a mobile app,

111

a glass jar with a plant, an irrigator, a light bulb and sensors. The wearable device uses pulse and light sensors to check whether you're engaging in positive daily activities such as taking in a healthy amount of sunshine or breathing in clean air in an open space. If you pass the test, the app will release water and food to the plant.

In the words of the team: "If the user takes the total healthy dose of sunlight for her body, the plant will also receive the light it needs for its growth. If the user visits two open space leisure places per week, the plant will also receive during the course of the week the nutrients it needs. This relationship of the plant with the user creates an emotional link, making her change her daily habits so her Symbio can survive. If the user keeps herself healthy, she will automatically keep the plant healthy."

Now there's an incentive to take the stairs instead of the elevator.

Coming to your senses: meditation

The practice of meditation stands outside biophilia and environmental psychology, yet it seems to be so obviously relevant to everything in this book. The state of mind it produces is very close to the way we often feel when we're focused on nature, a feeling which can only be enhanced by mindful and conscious awareness of the moment.

In the autumn of 2013 I decided to learn mindfulness meditation. Years before, I had enjoyed reading 'Zen Computer', a light-hearted spiritual guide for the wired user, in which the author Philip Toshio Sudo advises: 'Don't ask where the path is. You're on it.' In that spirit, I decided to try two different paths for my explorations: Insight Timer, a smartphone app which maps and connects fellow meditators across the world, and The Buddhist Geeks, an online community producing podcasts about dharma, technology, and culture.[xlix] For both, the chosen spot for contemplation wasn't a temple or a church hall or a sitting room, but cyberspace.

Insight Timer can be used in a number of ways. At the simplest level, you set the timer and get started on your own. Alternatively, you can choose from a large number of guided meditations. Not only will it log your meditations in a tidy graph, but every time you start a session you appear as another yellow star on its little world map. On my first day, I learned that I was meditating alongside 438 other people across the world. Although it was impossible to pick out individuals, I could see that my fellow meditators were in the US, Europe, down the coast of China, in Australia, and in Africa. I used the app at home most of the time, but occasionally listened with earbuds at a quiet spot outdoors.

So how does it feel to meditate with invisible people? If you have spent a lot of time in virtual worlds, gaming online, or even just chatting in Facebook, you'll know that there can often be a strong sense of co-presence. I've also felt that

114

connection while spending time 'on the cushion' next to others in the virtual space of Insight Timer. It's not so much a sense of connecting with individual people, but more of a mind-meld moment with everyone involved.

Working with the Buddhist Geeks turned out to be intimate in a different way from Insight Timer. At the daily Open Practice sessions, we switched on our webcams and logged into Google Hangout to meditate in small groups. Each thirty minute session was usually attended by around half a dozen members. At the scheduled time we logged in one by one, greeted the others with a smile or hello, then someone quietly tapped a bell and we settled down to our individual meditations.

We sat together but not together. Sometimes we turned off our microphones to avoid making distracting noises, sometimes we kept them on and listened to each other breathing. We were thousands of miles apart, sitting in front of computers, tablets or phones, logged in from homes, offices and gardens. Although we were in

115

different countries and time zones, I somehow felt very close to my companions. We were side by side on the path, being mindful in cyberspace. In many ways it wasn't very different from the physical meditation meetings where I had shared similar silences.

My experiences of online meditation have made me wonder whether, if we can be together like this in virtual space, can mindfulness be extended to cyborgian or machine space? In other words, rather than meditate *in* Google, might we some day meditate *with* Google? Imagine that: entering a mind-meld with the great consciousness which is Google itself.

There are many ways to learn mindful meditation and not enough space to detail them all here. As well as the paths described above, I also attended weekly meetings near my home, and followed the work of Jon Kabat-Zinn, founder of the Mindfulness-Based Stress Reduction (MBSR) course at the University of Massachusetts Medical

School. The programme came out of his experiences studying Buddhism and yoga, and focuses on the progressive acquisition of mindful awareness. Widely adopted by health professionals, it has been shown to help with a wide range of difficulties such as chronic pain, depression, anxiety, and drug addiction. Kabat-Zinn is well-known for his recommendation to 'cultivate mindfulness as if your life depended on it, which it surely does'.

The cerebral experience of mindful meditation fits well into geek culture. Since 2007, Google has been offering its employees a mindfulness meditation course amusingly entitled 'Search Inside Yourself', and in recent years many other technology companies have started providing similar perks. For instance, Marc Benioff, the CEO of Salesforce, is a keen meditator, and his company HQ in San Francisco has a dedicated meditation room on each floor. The design was inspired by a group of Buddhist monks who had visited the old Salesforce offices and were very concerned about the intense levels of activity: 'Everywhere we go, everybody's talking all the time, they are working all the time, you got to stop this', they told him. Now, says Benioff, the quiet zones enhance creative innovation. 'employees can put their phones into a basket or whatever, and go into an area where there is quietness.'[1]

Meditation also fits well with another of the Kaplans' restorative experiences: 'compatibility'. This is about finding a setting which suits you personally. 'An environment may offer fascination and extent and still fall short as a setting for restorative experiences', say the Kaplans. In other words, a situation might seem to offer all the required benefits yet still not work for you. Or maybe it doesn't allow you to follow the activity you would prefer. Meditation can address this possibility of discomfort because it allows the user to deal with the limitations of the physical by opening up the virtual space of the mind. I've meditated in places which offer little compatibility, but found myself able to be mentally transported to a mountain, a lake, or even high amongst the stars. In other words, just because a place is biophilic doesn't mean it's *your kind* of biophilic.

Nearby nature

When I was writing *Technobiophilia: nature and cyberspace* I lived for a while in a cottage in a rural part of the English Midlands. My desk stood in front of a window which overlooked a small courtyard containing potted plants. I had arranged the pots so they looked good when you were outside, but from indoors you could only see a few of them. Most of the time, they lay just outside my line of sight.

This meant that when I was working at my desk, which was for a good number of hours each day since the art of the writer involves applying the seat of the pants to the seat of a chair, the view beyond the lid of my laptop consisted only of one single plant: a deciduous white clematis which bloomed gloriously for a few months and looked like a clump of dead sticks the rest of the time. But I was so deep in my work that I didn't even notice what I was missing.

I lived in that cottage for two years, and it was twelve months before it suddenly dawned on me that most of the greenery I had spent money and time on was at the other end of the courtyard and invisible from my window. While I was sitting writing about the importance of nature, I was totally neglecting my own wellbeing. I felt rather foolish when I realised that not only would a simple rearrangement of the pots bring colour and foliage into my view all day long, they would also be a working application of the biophilic sensibility I was thinking about day after day. Epic fail.

I ran outside and lugged the pots across the courtyard until they were in the right location. After that, when I worked at my desk I could raise my eyes from the screen and enjoy brilliant red geraniums blooming for months, multi-coloured mesembryanthemums opening to the sun, and a succession of other beautiful and renewing greenery.

In the 1980s, experimental psychologists Rachel and Stephen Kaplan found that these kinds of small glimpses of the natural world, which they called *'nearby nature'*, could have powerful and measurable effects.

Instances of nearby nature are small suggestions of the natural world which, although seemingly insignificant and often out of physical reach, can play an important role in human wellbeing. Even the sight of a few trees viewed through a window can provide a sense of satisfaction, and people with acccss to nearby natural settings have been found to be healthier than those without. Studies show they experience increased levels of satisfaction with their home, job and life in general.[li]

I was especially interested to learn that nearby nature doesn't have to be beautiful or complex, and you don't even have to be physically close to it to gain the benefits. The Kaplans found that it's just as potent when viewed through a closed window or seen pictorially via a photograph, painting, video, or even something as mundane as a wall calendar.

In fact, it turns out that even my single woody clematis would have awarded me some kind of small benefit, if only I had thought to pay attention to it.

How we spend our days

Work/life balance used to be about how you divide your time. Should you focus on earning money and developing a career, or on family, health, spirituality and pleasure? Today, however, the ways we make a living are changing. These days, work and life intersect more than they did fifty years ago.

Rather than be tied to the office, factory or shop, many of us are able to work more flexibly. Some companies have adopted agile forms of organisation, where employees choose where, when and how to work. This way, our daily

122

schedules can fit better with personal and family demands, operate across time zones, or suit a nomadic lifestyle. For an increasing number of us, regular working hours have become a distant memory and, while this is problematic for some, it has brought new kinds of freedom to others. More and more, work and life are becoming intertwined, just as they were before the Industrial Revolution.

In Europe before about 1800, there was little differentiation between work and life. Work *was* life in an agrarian handicraft economy where people grew and made most of what they needed, and time was shaped by seasonal and cultural calendars. But as soon as steam-powered machines were invented, and the spinning-wheel was superseded by the power loom, automated production could run 24/7. Workers had to keep up, and soon the factory day became the norm.

Now, the Information Revolution has triggered another change. In the twenty-first century, we're learning to adjust as the ecosystem of labour evolves yet again. A hundred years ago, workers feared being treated as if they were robots; today they fear being replaced by robots. In fact the future of employment is not all about robots - it's much more complicated than that - but the nature of work is certainly changing rapidly. The 'traditional' workday is becoming shorter, sometimes more fragmented, and definitely more entwined with the rest of our waking hours. And even the very nature of our labour, of what we actually do all day, is being transformed too. Perhaps some of us will even make a healthy income from going back in time and returning to the spinning wheel. After all, handmade goods are the new luxury products.

There are many possibilities. But one thing we're coming to understand, better than ever before, is the importance of wellbeing in whichever lifestyle we choose. We're beginning to realise that, to paraphrase the poet Annie Dillard, the way we spend our days is the way we spend our lives.

Tech/nature balance

How can we maintain a healthy balance between our lives in technology and our lives in nature? This issue reflects some of the challenges as the work/life balance, so I've called it the *tech/nature balance*.

The problem goes like this: many of us are connected to the internet pretty much all the time. It's where we work, where we play, where we meet up with people and stay in touch with distant friends and family, and that's fine. But there's something else we could be connecting to that has rather fallen by the wayside: Planet Earth. The soil beneath our feet. The air we breathe. The forests, beaches, fields, mountains, lakes and gardens of the natural world.

Today, most of us live in cities which are not exactly rich in greenery. In the 1800s, millions of rural workers migrated to the cities and became urbanites. They got used to buying their food instead of growing it, and there was no longer any opportunity to keep their own livestock for eggs and meat. They could still make their own clothes, but before long it was cheaper to buy them off-the-peg. That kind of lifestyle became just a sentimental memory, although of course the reality of rural life is tough and not at all romantic.

Have we lost touch with nature? Many feel we have. At first we blamed it on the factories, then the car, then the TV, and now we blame it on the internet. But that's incorrect.

It's *we* who are responsible.

We came to believe that we could concrete over the fields and design a better life for ourselves, free of nature's wildness and uncertainties. But it's very obvious now that this was the wrong way to go.

We need to develop a different kind of balance, a tech/nature balance. One which helps us live more healthily in cities and more naturally with our technology.

Many people are already doing this. They are

finding ways to integrate their online lives with the physical world of nature and the outdoors. Others are getting their daily dose of nearby nature online or using social media to organise and support their outdoor lives. There are all kinds of ways to bring nature and technology together to improve health and wellbeing. Some are obvious, others less so.

This revolution affects us all. It's important for everyone, but particular groups like children, seniors, and people with medical issues or disabilities will gain particular benefit from its influence. And the concept of tech/nature balance is important in conversations about health, sustainability and the environment, biomimicry and design, architecture and planning.

It's impossible to cover all these topics in this small book, but the ideas are very transferable and I hope that Part 3 will help you make a start.

There are many ways to work towards a better tech/nature balance. In Part 3 I've collected 50 tips, tricks and experiments to try for yourself. Enjoy, share your favourites, and let me know how you get on!

3. Putting it into practice

*'Just as we go into a redwood grove and get that
cathedral-like feeling, I think that as the internet
continues to complexify and become larger, it will
also become a spiritual place where people will
retreat to feel something bigger than themselves'.*

(Kevin Kelly)

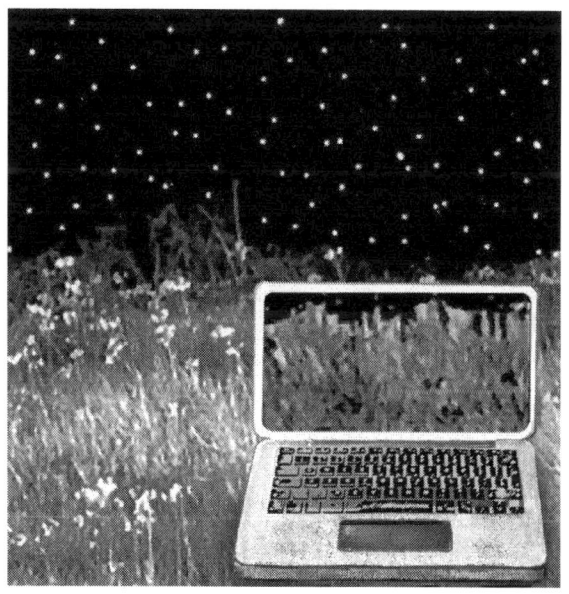

Audit your tech/nature balance

Let's start with an informal audit of your own tech/nature balance. How many of the following have you done in the last seven days?

Group A	Group B
☐ Felt bare earth with your fingers? ☐ Eaten a raw fruit or vegetable? ☐ Tended a plant? ☐ Made skin contact with living wood? ☐ Gazed at the sky for over a minute? ☐ Touched a live animal? ☐ Swum in open water - sea, river, lake? ☐ Walked in a green place? ☐ Touched natural stone or rock? ☐ Spent time near water?	☐ Touched a computer keyboard? ☐ Spoken on a phone? ☐ Played a video game? ☐ Spent time on Facebook? ☐ Tweeted? ☐ Taken a digital photo? ☐ Recorded or watched a digital movie? ☐ Skyped or FaceTimed? ☐ Sent a text message? ☐ Watched TV ?
TOTAL	TOTAL.....

How does your score for Group A compare with

that for Group B? Does the result surprise you? Do you need to make any changes to your day? Perhaps the following pages will help you find a few things you'd enjoy doing. Give them a try, and share your favourites.

Dip in and out as you please. Some will appeal to you, others not. If you devise your own tips and tricks, please share them too.

50 tips, tricks and experiments to try

1. What can you see from your window? If nothing much, consider moving the furniture or changing the position of greenery inside and out. Small alterations can make a huge difference to the availability of nearby nature.

2. If you're unlucky enough to have no windows in your room or workspace, consider creating faux views with pictures, screens, and plants. There's evidence that these kinds of images can reduce stress.

3. Choose more nature, not less technology. Set your timer for 2 minutes, lift your gaze from your screen, and watch the sky until the timer goes off.

4. Don't log off if you don't want to. But if you do, do. Look out for differences in how you

feel when you're online or offline.

5. When you're browsing through Facebook, Twitter or anywhere else on the web, take time to stop and appreciate other peoples' nature photos. They can be spectacular. Look out for breath-taking sunrises, evocative dusks, gorgeous landscapes and intoxicating blooms The best sites to create albums of your own and others' choice images are Pinterest and Instagram.

6. Don't let people make you feel anxious or guilty about the pleasure you get from being online, using your phone, or messing around on your tablet. You live in the twenty-first century! Enjoy your wired life!

7. Choose a day when you can commit to noticing your encounters with nature, both real and virtual, and keep notes about your experiences. Repeat favourites and try new

ones. Saunter through the countryside and get muddy. Wander through the wilderness in a video game. Notice how many times you 'like' other peoples' nature photos, or they 'like' yours. If you're keeping a journal, make a note of these interactions and how they make you feel.

8. Vinyl wall stickers, or decals, can transform a space, especially if teamed with natural plants. I have a floor-to-ceiling decal of a leafy tree, and in front of it a real and wildly flourishing swiss cheese plant. Together they look fantastic!

9. Get to know the forest through the senses of another creature. 'In the eyes of the animal' is a virtual reality 360 experience by Marshmallow Laser Feast. Billed as 'a journey through the food chain', it's an artistic interpretation of the sensory perspectives of three British species. New

135

Scientist described it as 'reality beyond our human limits'.

10. Ignore instructions to leave your kit at home. Take it with you whenever you feel like it. It's up to you whether you decide to use it, or not.

11. Stream the outdoors to the indoors via the web or TV. Some channels show 'slow TV', hours-long live programmes of countryside or waterscapes. Track live webcams of landscapes, birds and animals all around the globe.

12. Sharpen your senses. Beneath your level of awareness, your biophilic memory could be picking up long-forgotten smells, tastes, sounds and sensations of the world. They may have been there since childhood. For me, the list includes the warm odours of a hen-house; the intense perfume of

greenhouse tomatoes; white dog-roses; anything to do with the beach; the scent and feel of cool grass in a sunny park. Find them, recognise them, remember them. Bring them to the surface.

13. When you're looking for a new screen wallpaper, consider a forest. Research has shown that pictures of dense groups of leafy trees are very calming.

14. Experiment with forest bathing, online or offline.

15. Audit your workplace. How does it rate for nature benefits?

16. Choose nature images for your desktop wallpapers and screensavers and make sure you spend a few minutes actually looking at them now and again. Use images that speak to you. Maybe you would prefer

137

the close-up of a sunflower you took last year on holiday to a stunning stock photo of a tropical island. Or maybe not. Biophilia operates mostly in the subconscious, so go with your gut preferences.

17. Learn a new digital skill on your smartphone or tablet. You're never too old to take a photo, record sound, identify a flower, or join a special interest group online.

18. If you like a geeky approach to gardening, try hydroponics. It's a method of growing plants using mineral nutrient solutions, in water, without soil, or sometimes in an inert medium like perlite or gravel. Plenty of opportunities for messing around with intriguing components and, hopefully, producing something edible or beautiful, or both.

19. Bring some plants into your workplace if

that's allowed. Position them where they can be seen and enjoyed. Look after them properly.

20. Keep a journal of your place in the natural world as you move through it every day. Draw maps. Notice the trees, plants and animals in your neighbourhood.

21. What part do animals play in your life? If you own a dog, cat, horse, or other animal, spend your time with them mindfully. If you have no animals nearby, consider bringing them into your home and workplace in the form of pictures, sculpture and design. Images and shapes of animals and other creatures, used in the patterns of curtains and rugs for example, are thought to reduce stress levels.

22. Take a trip into virtual reality to explore VR forests, plains, deserts, and oceans. Try

video games too. Second Life has a wealth of landscapes to enjoy, and the mountains in Grand Theft Auto are stunningly beautiful all year round. Treat yourself to a cheap Google Cardboard kit or a fancy VR headset to open up whole new vistas. Be a VR tourist.

23. Choose a topic or activity to learn about this year - the shore, hedgerows, birds - and take your smartphone with you. There are lots of apps especially created for the outdoors, many of which work even when you can't get a signal.

24. Pay attention to the sounds of nature – birdsong, rustling leaves, weather. Find them in the digital too. There are numerous apps of birdsong, and many recordings of the weather to listen to. I know someone who does his best thinking when rainfall is playing on his phone. This year, 2017, BBC

Radio Three will live-stream the audio of twelve mile hike in the Black Mountains of Wales, from the village of Cwmdu across the mountains to Hay-on-Wye. It's expected to last for four hours, another example of slow broadcasting. Sound is a very effective way to access your hidden biophilic sensorium.

25. What might 'being away' mean for you? Are you aware of when you need it? Where do you go to 'be away'? Offline, online, both?

26. Share your pictures. Setting aside a moment to gaze and share can help soothe your connected life.

27. Have fun! The Buddhist Boot Camp shared of great photo of a man relaxing beside a fast-running river. 'Can I call you back?' he says to someone on his mobile. 'I'm watching a live stream.' And he really is.

28. De-stress your digital life with something made from real wood – perhaps a mouse, a keyboard, or a smartphone case.

29. Look up! Raise your eyes to the sky, the trees, the world. Simple, but so easily forgotten.

30. Look down! There are microcosms of nature beneath your feet. Do you ever think about them?

31. Are there any woodlands, forests or parks in your area? Plan to spend an hour or two amongst densely-packed trees, longer if you can. Walk, sit, relax. Open your senses.

32. Make something with your hands. Is it a long time since you did that? Remind yourself of the feel of clay, wood, cotton,

wool, metal, even paper. When you're outdoors, revive childhood pursuits like making daisy-chains, rosehip pigs, and twig catapults. Or experiment. Artist Andy Goldsworthy sewed leaves with thorns and used his own spit to stick icicles together. Pile some stones. Carve some wood. Make stuff.

33. Go outside without a purpose. Just wander about, loll around, with or without your phone. Wake up and smell the flowers.

34. How many natural materials do you physically touch every day - real wood, soil, leaves, flowers, and vegetables?

35. If you enjoy a bit of circuitry you might want to try connecting plants to networks. For example, the OrchGard project in Grimsby, received funding from the National Youth Agency to create a community digital

orchard/garden that will use the latest technology to keep the fully automated orchard as productive as possible. The project is based at the YMCA Humber in Grimsby. It aims to increase social cohesion and create awareness for the environment through the shared medium of digital technologies. A long-term venture worth watching.

36. No access to real plants in your workplace? Get yourself a virtual succulent from *Viridi*[lii]. According to its makers, it will keep you company while you work. Tending to it will, apparently, provide daily meditative moments.

37. Estimate how much your usual daily dose of nature might be. A ten minute walk to the bus-stop? Taking the dog out for half an hour? Can you plan to increase it over

time?

38. Green Exercise, sometimes called the Green Gym, is about taking exercise in natural environments – in other words, outdoors. It includes general exercise programmes as well as volunteer environmental restoration work like forestry, digging ditches, and other physical activity. Some programmes also offer forest bathing. Perhaps there's a Green Gym or outdoor volunteer programme near you.

39. Did you tend a plant today? Stroke an animal? Seek out a ray of sunlight and raise your face to its warmth?

40. Look around your home for ways to include biophilic design. Stone, wood, wool, natural fabrics - what do you have in the way of natural materials? Can you do something more interesting with the way you display

145

your plants?

41. Collect stones, wood, or shells. Clean and shape them yourself. Set aside time now and then to enjoy the feel of them in your hands – the surface, the weight, the coolness, the warmth.

42. If you like lists, there are lots of opportunities, and plenty of apps to use to record birds seen, plants grown, clouds and stars observed, walks taken, activities by day, by week, by month. You get the picture.

43. Do you need to be indoors all the time at work? Why not take your laptop outside, or hold your meetings there - in a park, on the beach, at the top of a mountain?

44. Indoor plants don't just promote wellbeing, they also clean the air. In 1989, NASA

conducted a now famous study into the best ways to clean the air in space stations. The result was a list of air-filtering varieties which don't just absorb carbon dioxide and release oxygen, as all plants do, but also eliminate significant amounts of benzene, formaldehyde and trichloroethylene. NASA researchers suggest using at least one plant per 100 square feet of space to clean the air effectively, an invaluable bonus in rooms stuffed with electronic equipment like laptops, printers and scanners. NASA especially recommends English ivy (Hedera helix); Peace lily (Spathiphyllum 'Mauna Loa'); Variegated snake plant, commonly known as Mother-In-law's tongue (Sansevieria trifasciata 'Laurentii'); Red-edged dracaena (Dracaena marginata) and Florist's chrysanthemum (Chrysanthemum morifolium).

45. If you want to geek out on technobiophilia,

try correlating your nature notes with data from your activity tracking software. Perhaps you could produce a technobiophilic data visualisation? Don't forget to share and compare the results.

46. If you want to increase your family's contact with nature but you're not very confident about your own knowledge, there are plenty of resources to help you. Richard Louv's book 'Vitamin N' is full of ideas. Or try the www.thewildnetwork.com, dedicated to helping you and your kids get more wild time. If you fancy an adventure, visit www.getoutwiththekids.co.uk.

47. Slow down. Just because the internet is fast doesn't mean you have to experience it at speed. We get anxious about rushing through our digital lives, but we don't need to be. Gaze at some pictures. Listen to

music. Build a beautiful website.

48. Make a resolution that you will:
    - connect with nature in a small way every day
    - spend at least one whole day a month outside
    - have a nature adventure once a year

49. Do you meditate? Perhaps you have thought about trying it. Today is always a good day to start.

50. Go for a walk :)

Afterword: an integrated life

'You didn't come into this world. You came out of it, like a wave from the ocean. You are not a stranger here.' (Alan Watts)

I hope this book has helped you feel optimistic about living well with nature in the digital age.

Connected life has brought many challenges, for sure, and sometimes it feels that the only way to deal with them is to turn your back and go fishing for trout in some rural retreat like the author I quoted in the Foreword.

But not only will running away not solve anything, it also deprives us of an array of glorious opportunities, many of which can't even be imagined yet. As long ago as 1991, the visionary computer scientist Mark Weiser wrote 'There's more information available at our fingertips during a walk in the woods than in any computer system, yet people find a walk among trees relaxing and

151

computers frustrating. Machines that fit the human environment, instead of forcing humans to enter theirs, will make using a computer as refreshing as taking a walk in the woods.'[liii] Are we closer to fulfilling his prediction? Perhaps.

For too long, urban life has been tearing us away from our heritage, our own planet, and the earth we walk upon. It may seem ironic that, in the end, technology will probably provide the tools we need to reconnect us with our biophilic sensibilities.

There will always be occasions when we want to leave technology behind completely, and others when it's good to embrace it. Equally, there are moments when our only desire is to immerse ourselves in skies and oceans and deserts, and others when we're comfortable at home surrounded by our material possessions.

For me, the discovery of technobiophilia has been a wake-up call and my life is richer for it. I hope yours is too.

I haven't been able to cover all the areas connected to this topic. The issue of children's relationships with nature and technology requires a separate book on its own, as do conversations about the elderly, the sick, and the disabled. There's no room here to do them justice but more will be written, I'm sure, in the years ahead.

I encourage you to create your own tech/nature recipes. Design a life which meets the needs of you, your family, and your community, one which responds to evolving preferences and situations.

Please don't succumb to pressure to curb your love of technology. Plan, instead, to expand your connections with the natural world. Nature, wellbeing and the digital life can be comfortable bedfellows if we choose to make them so. It's up to us.

I hope, too, that you feel optimistic about our digital future. Please share your stories about the issues I've raised here. Has anything changed for you since reading this book? Have you become more conscious of biophilia? Have you made efforts to improve your tech/nature balance? What works for you? What challenges do you face?

Today as I write this, I'm sitting on my tiny balcony, four floors up. It's crammed with plants I've battled to keep alive against the wild sea winds that blow in from the Channel.

In 'Moby Dick', Herman Melville described the ordinary citizens of a coastal town who like to spend their free time just gazing out to sea. 'Circumambulate the city of a dreamy Sabbath afternoon', he wrote. 'What do you see? – Posted like silent sentinels all around the town, stand thousands upon thousands of mortal men fixed in ocean reveries'.

What do those people feel connected to? Each other, for sure, but also to a sense of something more, something beyond.

I, too, am fixed in an ocean reverie. It's a clear bright day and I can see the golden sands and green hills of Purbeck ten miles away across the bay. To the west lies the bright whiteness of Old Harry Rocks and the curve of Swanage behind them. The sea between is a hundred shades of blue. The sky is scattered with white puffy clouds.

My laptop rests on the table before me. The sun warms my cheeks. I click the mouse.

The End

Share

Do you have thoughts or stories about digital wellbeing? I'd like to hear them.

Join me at the Digital Wellbeing Facebook Group
https://www.facebook.com/groups/digitalwellbeing

Tweet me
@suethomas

Check out my blog
www.suethomas.net

Other books by Sue Thomas
Technobiophilia: Nature and Cyberspace (2013)
Hello World: Travels in Virtuality (2004)
Wild Women (1994)
Water (1994)
Correspondence (1992)

Endnotes

---

[i] Boyle, Mark. 'No bills, so many riches: the lessons of living like a prince outside cyberia' The Guardian 6/2/17 https://www.theguardian.com/commentisfree/2017/feb/0 6/life-without-technology-tech

[ii] Gooley, T. How to Connect with Nature. Macmillan, 2014.

[iii] Abram, D. The Spell of the Sensuous, Vintage, New York, 1997.

[iv] Berry, W. 'Against PCs'. Harper's Magazine, September 1988.

[v] Liz Wagoner, Adjunct Professor at Kent State University

[vi] Urban green spaces and health. Copenhagen: WHO Regional Office for Europe, 2016. http://www.euro.who.int/__data/assets/pdf_file/0005/321 971/Urban-green-spaces-and-health-review-evidence.pdf

[vii] Beres, Damon. 'Reading On A Screen Before Bed Might Be Killing You' Huff Post. 30/11/15 http://www.huffingtonpost.com/2014/12/23/reading-before-bed_n_6372828.html

viii Wilson, E.O. 'Biophilia', 1984.

ix Monbiot, George. 'The primal thrill of sharks: the emotional case for rewilding the sea'. 4.2.17 The Guardian

x Ulrich, R.S. 'Human responses to vegetation and landscapes'. Landscape and Urban Planning Vol. 13, 1986: 29– 44, 29.

xi Kaplan R. and Kaplan, S. 'The Experience of Nature', Cambridge University Press, 1989.

xii See papers listed on the website of the Society of Forest Medicine. http://forest-medicine.com/page11.html

xiii Porter, Roy. 'Reading is Bad for your Health' History Today, 3.3.98 http://www.historytoday.com/roy-porter/reading-bad-your-health

xiv Greenfield, Susan. 'On Screen Technologies' n.d. http://www.susangreenfield.com/science/screen-technologies/

xv Roger S. Ulrich. 'View through a window may influence recovery from surgery'. Science Vol. 224 No. 4647, 27 April 1984: 420–421.

xvi Roger S. Ulrich. 'Biophilic theory and research for healthcare design'. In Biophilic Design, by Stephen R. Kellert, Judith R. Heerwagen and Martin L. Mador. New Jersey: John Wiley & Sons, 2008, 92.

[xvii] Roger S. Ulrich, Robert F. Simons, Barbara D. Losito, Evelyn Fiorito, Mark A. Miles, Michael Zelson, Stress recovery during exposure to natural and urban environments, Journal of Environmental Psychology, Volume 11, Issue 3, September 1991, Pages 201-230, ISSN 0272-4944, http://dx.doi.org/10.1016/S0272-4944(05)80184-7.

[xviii] 'Forest bathing'. Healthy Parks Healthy People. http:// www.hphpcentral.com/ article/ forest-bathing (accessed 15 December 2012

[xix] 'A Dose-Response Curve Describing the Relationship Between Urban Tree Cover Density and Self-Reported Stress Recovery' by Bin Jiang, Dongying Li, Linda Larsen, William C. Sullivan, Environment and Behaviour, Volume: 48 issue: 4, page(s): 607-629 DOI: https://doi.org/10.1177/0013916514552321 September 25, 2014

[xx] The Global Impact of Biophilic Design in the Workplace, Human Spaces, 2015.

[xxi] Health, Wellbeing & Productivity in Offices, The next chapter for green building. September 2014. The World Green Building Council.

[xxii] Popova, Maria. 'French Polymath Henri Poincaré on How Creativity Works' Brainpickings. n.d. https://www.brainpickings.org/2013/08/15/henri-

poincare-on-how-creativity-works/

[xxiii] Marc G. Berman, John Jonides and Stephen Kaplan. 'The cognitive benefits of interacting with nature'. Psychological Science Vol. 19 No. 12, 2008: 1207– 1212, 1211.

[xxiv] Gregory N. Bratman, Gretchen C. Daily, Benjamin J. Levy, James J. Gross, The benefits of nature experience: Improved affect and cognition, Landscape and Urban Planning, Volume 138, June 2015, Pages 41-50, ISSN 0169-2046, http://dx.doi.org/10.1016/j.landurbplan.2015.02.005.

[xxv] Thoreau, H.D. and Blaisdell, B. 'Thoreau's Book of Quotations', Dover.

[xxvi] Edward O. Wilson. Biophilia. Kindle. Cambridge: Harvard University Press, 1984, 139.

[xxvii] Paul Shepard. 'On animal friends'. In The Biophilia Hypothesis, by S. R. Kellert and E. O. Wilson, 275– 300. Washington: Island Press, 1993, 281– 282.

[xxviii] Stephen R. Kellert, 'Dimensions, elements and attributes of biophilic design'. In Biophilic Design, by Stephen R. Kellert, Judith H. Heerwagen and Martin L. Mador, 3. Hoboken: John Wiley, 2008,

[xxix] Beatley, Tim. 'The Technobiophilic City', Biophilic Cities Network. http://biophiliccities.org/the-

technobiophilic-city/

xxx Boxer, Sarah. 'Reading Proust on my cellphone', The Atlantic, June 2016. https://www.theatlantic.com/magazine/archive/2016/06/reading-proust-on-my-cellphone/480723/

xxxi Hinsliff, G. 'How living offline became the new status symbol'. The Guardian. 15 January 2016. https://www.theguardian.com/commentisfree/2016/jan/15/living-offline-status-symbol-eddie-redmayne

xxxii Jurgenson, N. 'The IRL fetish'. The New Inquiry. 28 June 2012 http://thenewinquiry.com/essays/the-irl-fetish/

xxxiii Adapted from Thomas, S. 'Nothing wrong with a digital detox but wired nature is better'. The Conversation. 19 March 2014 http://theconversation.com/nothing-wrong-with-a-digital-detox-but-wired-nature-is-better-24499

xxxiv 65Jennifer Van Grove. 'FarmVille users plant 310 million virtual organic blueberries'. Mashable. 22 July 2010. http://mashable.com/2010/07/22/farmville-organic-blueberries/

xxxv Thomas, Sue, "Gazing at Virtual Nature Is Good for Your Psychological Well-Being". Slate Magazine, December 2013. http://www.slate.com/blogs/future_tense/2013/12/17/nea

---

rby_nature_effect_biophilic_design_looking_at_virtual_tr
ees_is_good_for.html

xxxvi Nielsen, Holly, 'Why sentimental pastoral themes
make perfect fodder for video games'. The Guardian,
November 2016
https://www.theguardian.com/technology/2016/jan/11/wh
y-sentimental-pastoral-themes-make-perfect-fodder-for-
video-games

xxxvii Deltcho Valtchanov. 'Physiological and affective
responses to immersion in virtual reality: Effects of
nature and urban settings'. PhD Thesis, University of
Waterloo, Ontario, Canada, 2010.

xxxviii Hartmann, Patrick and Vanessa Apaolaza-Ibáñez.
'Virtual nature experiences'. Environment and Behavior
Vol. 40 No. 6, November 2008: 818– 842.

xxxix Thomas, Sue. Technobiophilia: Nature and
Cyberspace, Bloomsbury 2013, p38.

xl Every Room Has a View: An Inside Look at Quantum
of the Seas' Virtual Balconies, YouTube,
https://www.youtube.com/watch?v=4__AIB8BI-4

xli Downloadable from http://fc.umn.edu/

xlii Nicholls, Wallace J. Blue Mind, Little, Brown &
Company, 2014

xliii Benedict W. Wheeler, Mathew White, Will Stahl-

Timmins, Michael H. Depledge, Does living by the coast improve health and wellbeing?, Health & Place, Volume 18, Issue 5, September 2012, Pages 1198-1201, ISSN 1353-8292,
http://dx.doi.org/10.1016/j.healthplace201206015

xliv http://www.FeelReal.com

xlv The Virtual Human Interaction Lab, Stanford University,
https://vhil.stanford.edu/projects/2015/sustainable-behaviors/

xlvi Zuckerberg, Mark. Facebook post, 25.3.14
https://www.facebook.com/zuck/posts/10101319050523971

xlvii Monitor of Engagement with the Natural Environment: 2015 to 2016, Natural England.
https://www.gov.uk/government/statistics/monitor-of-engagement-with-the-natural-environment-2015-to-2016

xlviii Seeking Parks, Plazas and Spaces. The allure of biophilia in cities. (Terrapin Bright Green, 2016)

xlix Adapted from Thomas, Sue. 'Mass online meditation lets you zone out in cyberspace', The Conversation. 10.3.14 http://theconversation.com/mass-online-meditation-lets-you-zone-out-in-cyberspace-24052

---

[i] Kim, Eugene. 'Salesforce put a meditation room on every floor of its new tower because of Buddhist monks'. Business Insider. 7.3.16 http://uk.businessinsider.com/salesforce-put-a-meditation-room-on-every-floor-of-its-new-tower-2016-3?r=US&IR=T

[ii] Kaplan, R. and S. Kaplan. The Experience of Nature. Cambridge: Cambridge University Press, 1989.

[iii] http://store.steampowered.com/app/375950/

[iiii] Weiser, M. The Computer for the 21st Century. https://www.ics.uci.edu/~corps/phaseii/Weiser-Computer21stCentury-SciAm.pdf Thanks to Ivan Travkin for bringing this to my attention.

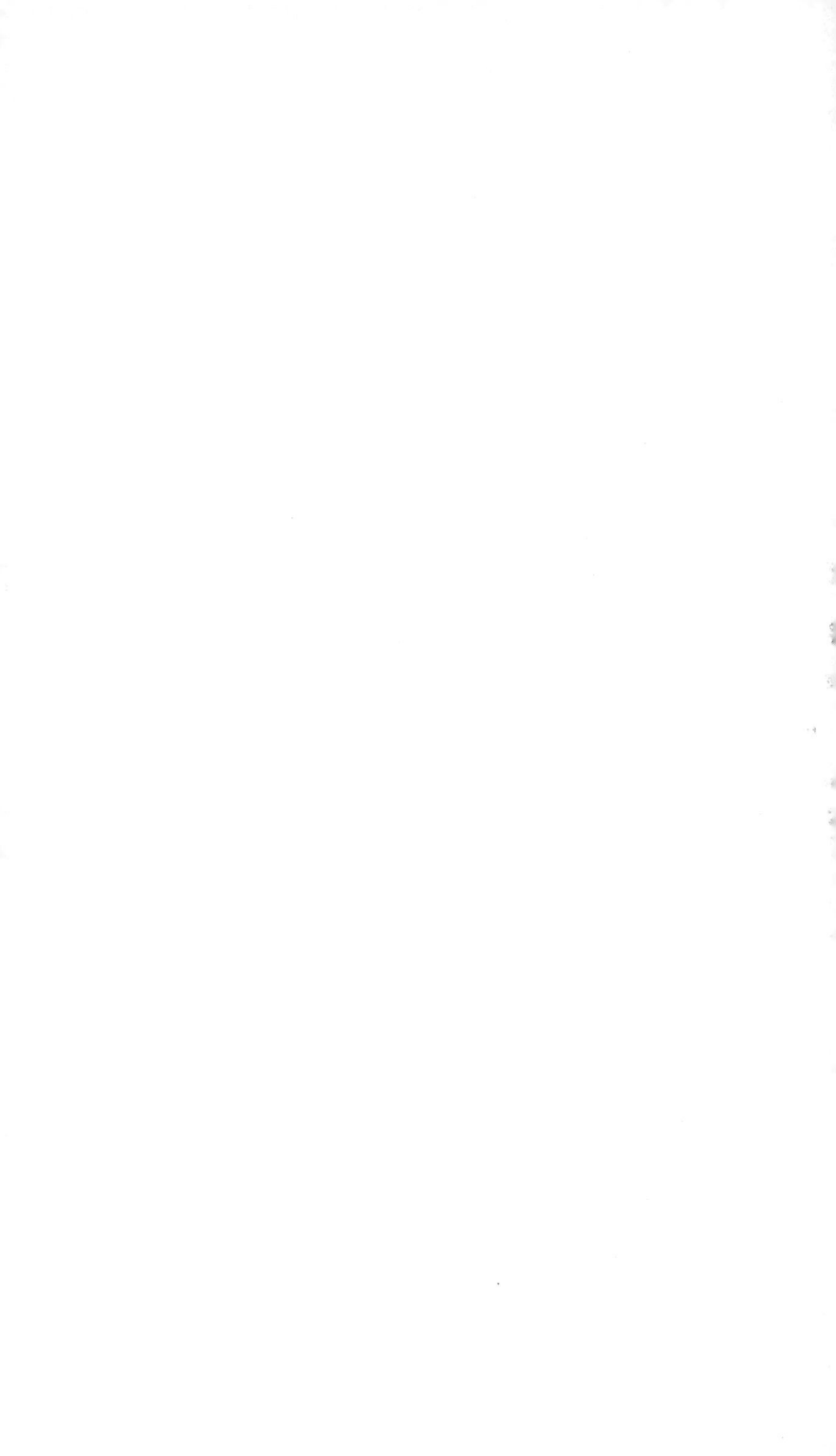

Printed in Poland
by Amazon Fulfillment
Poland Sp. z o.o., Wrocław